MYELOPROLIFERATIVE DISORDERS

SYMPTOMS, RISK FACTORS AND TREATMENT OPTIONS

RECENT ADVANCES IN HEMATOLOGY RESEARCH

MYELOPROLIFERATIVE DISORDERS

SYMPTOMS, RISK FACTORS AND TREATMENT OPTIONS

ANTHONY M. CAMDEN
EDITOR

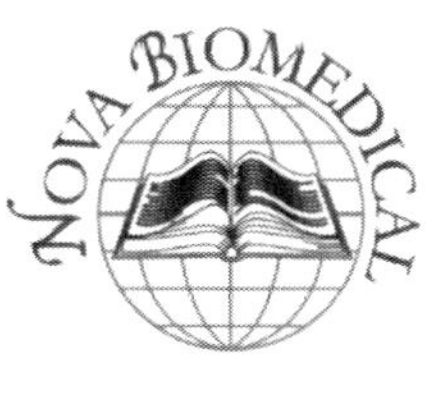

Nova Biomedical

New York

For permission to use material from this book please contact us:
Telephone 631-231-7269; Fax 631-231-8175
Web Site: http://www.novapublishers.com

NOTICE TO THE READER

Library of Congress Cataloging-in-Publication Data

ISBN: 978-1-63321-201-5
LCCN: 2014941660

Published by Nova Science Publishers, Inc. † New York

CONTENTS

PREFACE

Myeloproliferative disorders are a group of clonal haematological neoplasms characterised by proliferation of one or more cells of myeloid lineage. They are the result of acquired mutations in the progenitor cell leading to hyper proliferation or neoplastic expansion of more mature forms of myeloid cells. Cells retain their functional ability with some degree of defects and also lead to suppression of normal stem cells. The most common type of Myeloproliferative Neoplasms (MPN) can broadly be classified into BCR ABL positive (Chronic Myelogenous Leukemia) and BCR ABL negative Disorders (Polycythemia Vera PV, Essential Thrombocytosis ET and Primary Myelofibrosis PMF). There are other rare types which have relatively low incidence like chronic neutrophilic leukemia, chronic eosinophilic leukemia, systemic mastocytosis and myeloproliferative neoplasms unclassifiable. These are the indolent type of haematological malignancies associated with marrow hypercellularity and organomegaly, with gradual progression to myelofibrosis or transformation to acute leukemias. During the dormant course of the BCR ABL negative MPN, they are more prone to thrombo-hemorrhagic complications and the treatment strategy is directed mostly to prevent complications. The past decade; therapies for BCR ABL positive disease (CML) have been a milestone achievement in keeping the disease in remission for many years, preventing major complications and halting the progression of the disease. This book discusses the classification, diagnosis and treatment of myeloproliferative diseases and provides insight on the symptoms and risk factors involved in the diseases.

Chapter 1 - The Chronic myeloid leukemia (CML) is a clonal stem disorder characterized by marked proliferation of myeloid cell lineage in all stages of differentiation. CML is the most common, extensively studied myeloproliferative neoplasm with significant expansion of granulocytes and their precursors in the blood. It was first described in the beginning of 19th century and tremendous research was focused at clinical and molecular level, leading to better understanding of the pathogenesis of the disease and development of treatment modalities.

Chapter 2 - Myeloproliferative neoplasms (MPNs) are diseases in which clonal cells of one or more myeloid lineages proliferate in the bone marrow. Elevated megakaryopoeisis is prominent among these disorders and contributes to essential thrombocythemia, primary myelofibrosis, polycythemia vera, and chronic myelogenous leukemia, which are considered the most common MPNs. Acute megakaryoblastic leukemia is also characterized by expansion of the megarkaryocytic lineage. The diseases all share a similar clinical course, often exhibiting splenomegaly, hepatomegaly, thrombocytosis, and various clotting and bleeding symptoms. The similarity of symptoms necessitates a combination of histological, clinical, and cytogenetic tests in order to make an accurate diagnosis. The V617 JAK2 mutation has been identified in most patients with polycythemia vera, and is also present in a subset of patients with essential thrombocythemia and primary myelofibrosis. Novel mutations are also being studied for their relevance to the pathogenesis of MPNs and may allow for further differentiation of the diseases. However, bone marrow histopathology may still serve as the most discriminating method to diagnose these disorders. The MPNs all display distinct megakaryocyte morphology and the bone marrow histopathology allows for investigation of proliferation of other hematopoietic lineages.

Chapter 3 - Janus-activated kinase 2 *(JAK2)* translocations have been described in hematologic malignancies involving both lymphoid and myeloid lineages. Better characterized translocation partners are *ETV6/TEL* on chromosome 12, *BCR* on chromosome 22 and the autoantigen Pericentriolar material-1 *(PCM1)* on chromosome 8. *PCM1-JAK2* fusion events are extremely rare and, to the authors' best knowledge, less than 30 clinical cases have been reported so far in the literature. Although the clinical onset of these disorders is extremely heterogeneous, several cases present with a myelodysplastic/ myeloproliferative disease with striking dysplastic features of the erythroid compartment.

Although recent studies showed an activation of the JAK/STAT axis in a *PCM1-JAK2*-transformed murine fibroblast or human lymphoma cell lines, little is known about signaling in primary cells from *PCM1-JAK2* patients. This aspect is extremely relevant if we consider the availability of new drugs targeting the JAK/STAT pathway (i.e. ruxolitinib).

The authors' group has recently studied the signaling pathways potentially activated by the PCM1-JAK2 chimeric protein in a patient harboring the rare translocation t(8;9)(p22;24), demonstrating that the ERK1/2 pathway is the signaling cascade primarily activated in *PCM1-JAK2* patient's neoplastic cells.

In this chapter, the authors will review the main aspects of *PCM1-JAK2-*related myeloid malignancies focusing on the newest biological insights and their implication for therapy.

Chapter 4 - The myeloproliferative neoplasms (MPN) are hematological diseases characterized by a myelo accumulation and clonal myeloproliferation of mature myeloid cells, which means peripheral blood granulocytosis, erythrocytosis and thrombocytosis.

The World Health Organization (WHO), in 2008, revised the criteria for classification and diagnosis of chronic myeloid neoplasms and now the Myeloproliferative Neoplasms (MPN) category includes chronic myelogenous leukemia (CML), polycythemia vera (PV), essential thrombocythemia (ET), primary myelofibrosis (PMF), chronic neutrophilic leukemia (CNL), chronic eosinophilic leukemia not otherwise categorized, hypereosinophilic syndrome (HES), mast cell disease (MCD) and MPN unclassified. This chapter will focus on diagnosis criteria, symptoms, risk factors and treatment options of myeloproliferative neoplasms, specifically CML, PV, and PMF.

The CML diagnosis is based on blood counts (leukocytosis and frequently also thrombocytosis) and the presence of circulating immature granulocytes, from the metamyelocyte to the myeloblast, and basophilia. Splenomegaly may be detected in >50% of patients in the initial chronic phase (CP), but 50% of patients are asymptomatic. Diagnosis is finally obtained by the observation of the Philadelphia (Ph) chromosome (22q-) and/or the *BCR-ABL1* oncogene in peripheral blood or bone marrow cells. CML is a tryphasic disease and the prognostic scores (Sokal and Hasford) were calculated based on patiens´age, spleen size and blood cell counts. Other patient characteristics must be considered in CML risk groups with a different prognosis, such as a different response rate, a different progression-free survival and a different overall survival, also for patients treated with imatinib. CML treatments currently used are hydroxyurea, tyrosine-quinase inhibitors (imatinib, dasatinib and nilotinib) and bone marrow transplantation. The WHO diagnostic criteria for the classic *BCR-ABL*-negative diseases, PV, ET and PMF, were based on cell myeloproliferation, morphologic and cytochemical features in bone marrow (biopsy and myelogram) as well as molecular findings (JAK2 and MPL mutations). In addition, other criteria are required for distinguishing the MPN subtypes for patients negative for JAK2 mutation. PV and ET patients present a high risk of thrombosis and a late risk of clonal evolution into PMF or acute myeloid leukemia (AML). PMF patients may also present a high risk of progressing to AML. The relations among laboratorial or molecular data and clinical features have been extensively studied and, as a consequence, the risk stratification, the risk-adapted therapy definition and systems for prognosis prediction have been improved for MPN patients. Besides the description of relative efficacy of many unspecific drugs for MPN, the molecular mechanisms discovery has made the development of target therapy with tyrosine kinases inhibitors possible. Many of them are in the final phase of clinical studies and some are already in clinical use.

In: Myeloproliferative Disorders
Editor: Anthony M. Camden

ISBN: 978-1-63321-201-5
© 2014 Nova Science Publishers, Inc.

Chapter 1

MYELOPROLIFERATIVE DISEASES: CLASSIFICATION, DIAGNOSIS AND TREATMENT

Farhan Mohammad[1], F. N. U. Vikram, M.D.[2],
Wajeeha Saeed, MD[3], George Everett, M.D.[2],
Amar Lal, M.D.[4],
*and Muhammad Rizwan Sardar, M.D.[5,6]**
[1]Staten Island University Hospital, Staten Island, NY, US
[2]Florida Hospital, Orlando, FL,US
[3]Albert Einstein College of Medicine, Bronx, NY, US
[4]Johns Hopkins International, Tawam Hospital, Abu Dhabi, UAE
[5]Lankenau Medical Center, Wynnewood, PA, US
[6]Thomas Jefferson University, Philadelphia, PA, US

CHRONIC MYELOID LEUKEMIA (CML)

The Chronic myeloid leukemia (CML) is a clonal stem disorder characterized by marked proliferation of myeloid cell lineage in all stages of differentiation [1]. CML is the most common, extensively studied

---

* Corresponding & senior author: Muhammad Rizwan Sardar, MD, Lankenau Medical Center, Thomas Jefferson University, 100 E Lancaster Avenue, Wynnewood, PA 19096; rizwansardar@hotmail.com; Tel: 347-327-2734.

myeloproliferative neoplasm with significant expansion of granulocytes and their precursors in the blood. It was first described in the beginning of 19th century and tremendous research was focused at clinical and molecular level, leading to better understanding of the pathogenesis of the disease and development of treatment modalities.

History and Epidemiology

Bennett proposed the theory of extreme pyemia, when he found enormous concentrations of leucocytes and splenic enlargement during autopsy results, but soon it was challenged by Virchow [2, 3, 4] and introduced the term 'leukamie (leukemia). Later, Neumann hypothesized that marrow is the site of leukemic cell production along with normal cells and coined the term myelogene (myelogenous) leukemia [5]. In 1960, Nowell and Hungerford discovered the presence of an abnormal chromosome in two patients and was designated as Philadelphia chromosome and this was the first time, a chromosomal abnormality was found in any human cancer [6]. A decade later, with the introduction of chromosomal banding techniques, the chromosomal abnormality was found to be a translocation between chromosome 9 and chromosome 22 t(9;22) [7]. The proto-oncogene ABL on chromosome 9 fuses with breakpoint cluster region (BCR) on chromosome 22 as a result of translocation resulting in the formation of fusion gene (BCR-ABL) [8, 9, 10, 11]. The gene encodes for a protein, which is a chimeric protein molecule of molecular weight 210,000 (p210) and has tyrosine kinase activity. P210 molecule is over expressed in cells obtained from patients with CML and is widely considered as the proximate cause of malignant transformation [12, 13, 14].

Around 5000 new cases of CML are diagnosed each year in United States and accounts for 15% of all leukemias and less than 5% of all childhood leukemias. There is increased incidence with age and peak age of incidence is in fifties. Men are more often affected than women. [15, 16].

Pathogenesis

The Philadelphia chromosome (Phl Chromosome) is the hallmark of CML and acquisition of Ph chromosome leads to molecular and cellular defects that ultimately lead to development of CML [6]. The acquisition of the defective chromosome occurs in a very early and primitive pluripotent stem cell. The genetically unstable cells have an abnormal growth pattern over normal stem cells and are characterized by unstable and uninterrupted proliferation of marrow elements predominantly myeloid precursors.

The trigger for the initiation of events is unclear and is not considered genetic as there is no correlation observed with monozygotic twins, geography or ethnicity. Prior exposure to radiation could possibly be one of the factors for the trigger as large number of events was reported from Nagasaki and Hiroshima [17]. BCR and ABL are normal proteins expressed in all the cells of an individual, on chromosome 22 and chromosome 9 respectively. In genetically unstable stem cell, there is a reciprocal translocation of the genetic material moving the 3' portion of ABL gene from chromosome 9 next to 5' portion of BCL gene, forming the BCR –ABL fusion gene on chromosome 22 [18]. The fusion occurs at distinct regions of the genes and breakpoint in the BCR determines the characteristics of the disease. There are three different regions in the BCR gene that have been described as major (M bcr), minor (m bcr) and mu bcr [19, 20, 21]. These regions have number of exons. Fusion occurs by translocation between one of the exons in BCR gene and second exon in ABL gene. If the breakpoint occurs in major region, the fusion leads to the formation of chimeric molecule and fusion oncoprotein with a molecular weight of 210kd (p210) and is the most common form seen in majority of CML cases. The m RNA transcripts of p210 oncoprotein have e14a2 or e 13a2 fusion junction of the translocation, where 'e' represents the BCR exon and 'a' represents ABL exon. If the breakpoint occurs in minor region, it leads to the formation of a smaller oncoprpotein p190 and is most commonly seen in Philadelphia positive ALL cases. If it occurs in the mu region, it forms a longer protein p230 [20, 21, 22, 23, 24].

The p210 (BCR-ABL) protein is located in the cytoplasm making it more accessible to a number of signal transduction pathways. A subunit of phosphotidylinositol kinase is associated with p210 and is responsible for proliferation of BCR ABL cell lines and CML cells. The fusion protein also inhibits apoptosis by delaying the M phase of the cell cycle [25].

Clinical Findings

The onset of symptoms in CML is gradual and most patients present in chronic phase. In today's medical practice, many patients are diagnosed even before they are symptomatic due to periodic medical examination. Fever, weight loss, bone pain, fatigue and left upper quadrant discomfort secondary to splenomegaly are the most common presenting symptoms [26, 27, 28]. Spleen size correlates with the leukocyte count and is rarely palpable with less than 40,000/mm3 leukocyte count. Hepatomegaly is less common. Very rarely, bleeding, thrombosis or leukemic infiltration of the skin or other organs may be the initial symptoms. Sternal tenderness is a reliable sign of disease and is limited to mid sternum.

Chronic phase eventually progresses to more advance stage of the disease called 'Blast Phase', characterized clinically by fever, night sweats, severe bone pain and refractory splenomegaly, which are markers of highly proliferative hematopoiesis. Extramedullary blastic chloromas are also seen. It has a high prevalence of central nervous system and lymph node chloromas. It is diagnosed on peripheral smear with greater than 20% blast cells with clumps of blasts cells. As the patient enters blast phase, other chromosomal abnormalities appear, in addition to Philadelphia chromosome. The progression to blast phase occurs at about 5% per year and increases to 20-25% each year thereafter [29, 30]. Patient suffers from all severe manifestations of acute leukemia like infection and hemorrhage. Once the blast phase is reached, the overall survival decreases to less than 6 months.

Sometimes, patients with chronic phase of CML may have worsening of the condition with hematologic deterioration and development of blasts cells, but less than 10% on peripheral smear. They are also characterized by increased leukocyte count, not responding to standard therapy. This phase is named 'Accelerated phase' of CML. Disease progression is identified by cytogenetic evolution and is often associated with appearance of second Philadelphia chromosome or trisomy 8 or iso-chromosome 17q [31, 32].

Diagnosis

A complete history and physical examination is a key to suspect CML. Presence of splenomegaly in a middle aged patient should always prompt ruling out CML.

A) *Blood*

A complete blood count with differential and peripheral smear examination should be the first initial step. Any degree of unexplained neutrophilic leukocytosis should prompt consideration of CML. Thrombocytosis is a common finding with very high platelet counts, but patient may not always present with this finding [33, 34]. An absolute basophilia is invariably present and is of extreme importance. Peripheral smear shows granulocytes in different stages of maturation with a characteristic 'bulge' on the myelocytic stage of maturation. Neutrophil alkaline phosphatase is low in 90% of patients with CML.

B) *Bone marrow*

All the myeloproliferative disorders are characterized by hypercellular marrow. In CML, myeloid to erythroid ratio is greater than 10 and blast cells are always less than 10%. Large numbers of small and 'dwarf' megakaryocytes are seen and are typical of CML [33, 35, 36]. However, a bone marrow biopsy is not always essential for making the diagnosis of CML and is often diagnosed with the detection of Philadelphia chromosome or BCR ABL fusion gene through cytogenetic and molecular studies.

C) *Cytogenetic Studies*

Cytogenetic analysis or karyotyping is done to identify the presence of Philadelphia chromosome. It can be performed ideally from the bone marrow material, but can also be done from the peripheral blood. The most common type of translocation in Philadelphia chromosome is t[9;22](q34;q11) and is present in more than 90% of the patients with CML. Less than 10% of the patients have variant translocations or cryptic translocations and are termed Philadelphia negative chromosomes. Variant translocations can involve translocation of 22q gene segment on to another chromosome other than 9 or translocations can involve more then two chromosomes [37, 38, 39]. It is difficult to identify Philadelphia negative chromosome with cytogenetic studies and needs FISH studies or PCR analysis.

D) *FISH (Fluorescent In Situ Hybridization) for BCR-ABL*

FISH helps in detection of location of BCR and ABL gene, when used with metaphase chromosomal preparations [40]. The specificity of FISH studies are greater in detection of complex chromosomal translocations compared to chromosomal banding. The interphase chromosomal preparations can also be used in both peripheral blood and bone marrow tissue, but has lower specificity compared to metaphase preparations.

E) *RT-PCR (Reverse Transcriptase-Polymerase Chain Reaction for BCR-ABL Fusion Gene)*

RT-PCR is the most sensitive method for detection of fusion protein because it uses the specific primers to amplify a DNA fragment from BCR ABL m RNA transcripts [41]. It is low cost and extremely sensitive that it can detect one Philadelphia chromosome in more than a million normal cells. It has now become test of choice in diagnosing CML and for monitoring treatment response and detects any residual disease after bone marrow transplantation.

Treatment

Therapy for CML depends on the phase of the disease. With the advent of tyrosine kinase inhibitors, patient achieve longer periods of remission and delay the progression of the disease. The treatment can broadly be classified in to three categories:

A) *Tyrosine kinase inhibitor's (TKI's)*

TKI's are the most effective and first line of treatment in chronic phase of CML. Imatinib is the first approved abl specific tyrosine kinase inhibitor and acts by inhibiting the BCR ABL-kinase activity and prevent the proliferation of Philadelphia positive CML cell lines [42]. Imatinib has achieved tremendous success in curtailing the progression of CML and achieving complete cytogenetic response. It helps in attaining complete hematologic response within 18 months of start of therapy. Studies have shown that at 5 years the cumulative incidence of complete cytogenetic response is about 75 percent and with estimated overall and progression free survival about 80 percent [43, 44]. Tyrosine Kinase Inhibitors (TKI's) are also used as first line therapy in 'accelerated phase' of CML.

The response to therapy in CML is assessed by hematologic, cytogenetic and molecular response criteria:

Hematologic response criteria: Complete hematologic response (CHR) is defined by a white blood cell count $<$ 10,000/microL with no immature granulocytes and $<$5 percent basophils on differential; platelet count $<$ 450,000/microL; and non palpable spleen [45].

Cytogenetic response criteria: Complete cytogenetic response is defined as no Philadelphia chromosomes identified, Major response with 1%-35% Philadelphia chromosomes, Minor Response with 36%-65% Philadelphia chromosomes, Minimal response with 66%-95% Philadelphia chromosomes and No response, if greater than 95% Philadelphia chromosomes identified in the marrow by chromosomal banding methods [46, 47].

Molecular response criteria: It is assessed by quantitatively measuring the cells through PCR method (Q-PCR). It is defined as log reduction below the baseline and can be less than 0.1%, 0.01% or 0.0032% on the international scale [46, 47].

Till date, there are five FDA approved TKI's in the market. Dasatinib, Nilotinib are second generation TKI's and are generally used in imatinib resistance. Studies are being done to look for the response rates when used as first line therapy instead of Imatinib. Bosutinib and Ponatinib has been recently approved for use in CML, not responsive to first and second generation TKI's [50, 51, 51, 53].

B) *Hematopoietic stem cell transplantation (HSCT)*

HSCT is the only curative treatment of CML, but due to its toxicity profile and adverse effects is less often opted by the patients. It is still the most effective therapy in young patients. After the introduction of TKI's, it is only used, when patients develop resistance to the standard therapy of TKI's. HSCT is best used in chronic phase of CML and good outcomes are obtained, if done within first year of diagnosis of the CML. The accelerated and blastic phase does not response well to HSCT and failure rate is greater than 85% [54, 55].

C) *Palliative chemotherapy*

Hydroxyurea, Busalfan, Interferon Alpha with or without Cytarabine and omacetaxine were commonly used before the discovery of TKI's. Hydroxyurea is still used in patients with high White count or High Platelet count, till the diagnosis of CML is established. It is used as a cytoreductive agent to decrease the counts and prevent the complications of thrombosis or bleeding. Prior to TKI's, Interferon alpha was used with or without cytorabine with cytogenetic response rate of around 10%-13%, but those who responded had a good survival rate(70%) at the end of 10 years.

Nowadays, it is only used only in patients who developed resistance or intolerant to TKI's. Toxicities with these combination drugs were greater and were replaced by TKI's [56, 57].

CHRONIC NEUTROPHILIC LEUKEMIA (CNL)

The Chronic neutrophilic leukemia (CNL) is a rare type of myeloproliferative neoplasm characterized by sustained elevation of mature clonal neutrophils with no immature granulocytes and not accompanied by basophilia or thrombocytosis. There is no molecular abnormality with CML, although few cases of presence of JAK2 mutation have been reported. Cytogenetic and molecular analyses are negative for Philadelphia chromosome and this is what differentiates it from CML. Leucocyte alkaline phosphatase is marked elvelated in CNL, but it is low in CML.

Clinically, CNL occurs in elderly individuals with a mean age of around 70 years and symptoms may consist of abdominal pain, anorexia, weakness, and easy bruising. It is associated with hepatosplenomegaly due to neutrophilic infiltration of the organs. Peripheral blood smear shows mature granulocytes without a left shift. Occasionally metamyelocytes, myelocytes and nucleated red blood cells may be seen. No blast cells or dysplastic features are seen. The bone marrow aspirate shows granulocytic hyperplasia with no increase in blast cells or any dysplastic features like hypogranulations are seen. Clinical course of CNL varies with some remaining stable for many years and others progressing with leukemic transformation. Median survival is 2-3 years. Interferon, Hydroxyurea and cytarabine have been tried, but long term benefits are unusual. Stem cell transplantation is the only curative option.

CNL is differentiated from a variant of CML called neutrophilic CML (CML-N) by the presence of Philadelphia chromosome a BCR-ABL fusion gene [58, 59, 60].

CHRONIC EOSINOPHILIC LEUKEMIA (CEL)

Typically in CEL, there is increase in eosinophil count with clonal proliferation of erythroid precursors. In the peripheral blood, there is marked increase in eosinophils with some premature forms and dysplastic features. Bone marrow is hypercellular with normal erythroid and myeloid precursors, but is packed with eosinophils and its precursors associated with dysplasia and blast cells. There is increase in blast cells although it is less than 20 percent.

Cytogenetic findings are common with high frequency of translocations. A molecular analysis shows an abnormal fusion gene present on chromosome 4 and is cryptic. Abnormal fusion gene involves PDGFRalpha and F1P1L1 gene is present. Patients who display this fusion gene respond well to Imatinib mesylate and may achieve long term remission [61, 62, 63].

CHRONIC MYELOMONOCYTIC LEUKEMIA (CMML)

Persistent monocytosis with dysplastic features and blast cells of less than 20 percent in the peripheral blood and bone marrow are characteristic of CMML and is differentiated from CML by the absence of Philadelphia chromosome. In CMML, more than 10% of monocytes are seen and rearrangements in PDGFRβ are seen and should be studied. Patient's positive for this gene can be treated with Imatinib mesylate. In the absence of this rearrangement, chemotherapy with cytarabine, hydroxyurea or etoposide can be tried with little success. In younger patients, the curative option would be allogeneic stem cell transplantation [64, 65].

POLYCYTHEMIA VERA (PV)

The Polycythemia Vera (PV) is a clonal stem cell disorder characterized by excessive proliferation of erythroid precursors that is part of pan myelosis in the bone marrow. There is trilineage proliferation of erythroid, myeloid and megakaryocytic cell lines, but mainly characterized by increased in red cell mass, erythrocytes and elevated hematocrit [66]. PV is clinically identified and distinguished from other MPN's by the presence of elevated red cell mass.

Polycythemia (increased red cell mass) can be broadly grouped into Primary Polycythemia (includes Polycythemia Vera rubra) and Secondary Polycythemia (Hypoxia related, Malignancy, Drug Associated). Relative Polycythemia is due to hemo-concentration secondary to dehydration, hypertension or Preeclampsia [67, 68]. In this chapter, only Primary polycythemia or Polycythemia vera (PV) are discussed in detail.

Epidemiology and Incidence

The median age at the time of diagnosis of PV is around 60 years. PV is a rare disorder occurring 0.6-1.6 per million populations and incidence is slightly higher in males. The true incidence could be higher, as many patients are asymptomatic and remain undiagnosed. Median survival in untreated patients of PV is 6-12 months, whereas with treatment the survival can exceed more than 10 years [66, 69].

Pathogenesis

PV is the most common primary polycythemia and is an acquired disorder resulting from a mutation in the bone marrow stem cell. JAK2 is present in all the hematopoietic cells and is necessary for proliferation of cells. The mutation in JAK2 V617F leads to unrestrained proliferation of erythroid precursors, irrespective of any response from hematopoietic growth factors. The extreme sensitivity to even small amounts of erythropoietin or in vitro proliferation of erythroid colony formation units without the addition of exogenous erythropoietin is the hallmark of PV [70, 71]. This mutation is identified in 95% of cases of Polycythemia Vera (PV). Five percent of cases are JAK2 V617F negative and could be the result of other mutations which still needs to be identified [72].

Clinical Features

PV can present with a variety of signs and symptoms and include headache, plethora, dizziness, pruritis, bleeding and thrombosis. But majority of patients are asymptomatic and diagnosed on periodic medical examination and elevated hemoglobin and RBC cell mass. Most of the symptoms are attributed to increased blood volume and red cell mass and are related to increased blood viscosity [67, 72, 73]. The lack of specificity of symptoms may delay the diagnosis.

Clinical Manifestation and Diagnosis

1) Skin Findings

Pruritis and Erythromelalgia are the two common skin findings associated with PV. Pruritis after a shower or bath is a common phenomenon and is present in 40% of the patients (also called aquagenic pruritis). It's attributed to release of histamine from the mast cells from the skin. Erythromelalgia is the burning pain, cyanosis (with palpable pulses) and erythema in the feet and hands associated with parasthesias [66, 73, 74, 75, 76]. These symptoms are related to microvascular thrombotic complications and are usually seen with high platelet count.

2) Thrombosis

Thrombosis is a major and most common complication of PV. Patients may present with a stroke, Myocardial Infarction, Pulmonary embolism or Deep Venous Thrombosis. Ten Percent of the patients can present with thrombosis of Hepatic Vein (Budd-Chiari Syndrome), which is a fatal complication. It can present with ascitis, abdominal pain, hepatosplenomegaly and jaundice, following the blockage of hepatic vein, hypoperfusion and necrosis of hepatocytes [66, 74, 77, 78, 79]. The association of Budd-Chiari Syndrome with PV is so strong, that any patient presenting with this syndrome should be evaluated for PV.

3) Bleeding

Although bleeding is a minor complication, some patients may present with easy bruising, gingival, nose bleeds or gastrointestinal bleeding [78]

4) Neurological Findings

Neurological symptoms are most related to thrombosis and may present with TIA's or Stroke. Visual disturbances or transient loss of vision can occur, which is secondary to hyperviscosity [77, 78].

5) Others

Pulmonary hypertension, pulmonary embolism, Myocardial Infarction, Angina, gout (due to high turnover of cells) and other vasomotor symptoms can be associated with PV [67, 73].

6) Natural History and Progression of Disease

Very late in the clinical course of PV, it can transform into myeloid metaplasia with myelofibrosis and acute leukemia. Post-polycythemia myelofibrosis or secondary myelofibrosis can be identified by development of anemia not related to iron deficiency, progressive increase in spleen size and marrow fibrosis [66, 71, 80, 81]. Extramedullary hematopoiesis takes place in spleen and liver causing hepatosplenomegaly. This phase is called 'spent' or 'burnt out' phase [82]. Development of spent phase is often associated with increased transformation to leukemic phase. Acute Leukemia as the terminal PV is invariable the fatal complication of the disease [82, 83, 84]. Although thrombotic complications still remain the leading cause of death in patients with PV.

7) Laboratory Findings

The complete blood count with a Hemoglobin/Hematocrit of 16.5/48 in women and 18/52 in men, associated with clinical impression of erythrocytosis should prompt the work up for polycythemia. Initially, it should be differentiated from spurious to true polycythemia and if it's true, whether it is primary or secondary. Primary polycythemia or Polycythemia vera can be diagnosed with the identification of JAK2 mutation and can be distinguished from reactive erythrocytosis.

The WHO criteria for the diagnosis of Polycythemia Vera includes the presence of two major and one minor criteria or presence of first major and two minor criterion: [86]

Major criteria	Minor criteria
1) Hemoglobin greater than 18.5 g/dl in men or 16.5 g/dl in women. 2) Presence of JAK 2 V617F mutation or any other functionally similar mutation.	1) Bone marrow biopsy showing hypercellularity with trilineage growth. 2) Serum erythropoietin below the reference range for normal. 3) Endogenous erythroid colony formation in vitro.

Peripheral blood: The hemoglobin, Hematocrit and Red blood cell mass are elevated in polycythemic stage of PV. Other Red blood cell indices are normal unless they are associated with other disorders. Red Blood Cells are normocytic, normochromic, associated with or without increase in Platelet count. The leukocyte cell lines from myeloid lineage can also be elevated. Secondary polycythemia can be differentiated from PV by the absence of thrombocytosis or basophilia, but it is not a definitive diagnostic indication.

Bone marrow: As mentioned in the minor criteria, bone marrow biopsy shows hypercellularity with proliferation of megakaryocytes and erythroid precursors [66, 69, 86]. In the modern era, after the discovery of JAK2 Mutation, Bone marrow biopsy is only performed only if the WHO criterion is not met through peripheral blood findings.

JAK2 mutation: Identification of JAK2 mutation is one of the major criteria and should be performed, if the diagnosis of PV is being considered. Ninety Five percent of the PV patients will have the mutation in exon 12 or exon 14 of this gene. Peripheral blood or bone marrow aspirate specimens can be used. It is very sensitive test and can detect a mutation, when present at 0.01 to 0.10% [66, 70, 71].

Serum erythropoietin: In PV, extreme erythrocytosis is associated with Low erythropoietin levels and suggests Red blood cell production is independent of erythropoietin levels or hypersensitive to erythropoietin levels and supports the diagnosis of PV. Erythrocytosis with high erythropoietin levels is very unlikely to be Polycythemia Vera and work up for the causes of secondary polycythemia should be initiated [66, 87, 88].

Endogenous erythroid colonies: This test is not routinely performed but almost all patients with PV have endogenous erythroid colonies [85, 89]. Bone marrow or peripheral blood cells, when grown invitro in a culture medium proliferate and form erythroid colonies in the absence of erythropoietin and these colonies are called "endogenous erythroid colonies".

Treatment

The primary goal of therapy in Polycythemia vera is to decrease the red cell count and prevent the complications associated with high erythrocyte count.

a. Phlebotomy: Phlebotomy is easily accessible, least expensive method of rapidly controlling the red blood cell count and bringing it to normal values. The only drawback is unable to control platelet and leukocyte count. It also does not prevent the major complication of Thrombosis in PV. Nevertheless, when combined with other agents, Phlebotomy is an excellent method of controlling the symptoms via decreasing the hematocrit. The target is to maintain the hematocrit of less than 45 [90, 91].

b. Hydroxyurea: The most widely used myelosuppressive agent in PV is Hydroxyurea and its efficacy in controlling erythrocyte, leukocyte and platelet count is well documented. Thrombotic complications are also less with hydroxyurea, when compared with phlebotomy alone. It rapidly decreases the platelet and leukocyte count and occasionally might need a phlebotomy to decrease the erythrocyte count [92, 93].

c. Anagrelide: It is a platelet aggregating agent and can be used to decrease the platelet count refractory to Hydroxyurea [94].

d. Anti Platelet agents: The thrombotic complications can be overcome with the use of Anti platelet agents like aspirin in high risk patients like age over 65 years and with history of an episode of thrombotic episode such as TIA, Myocardial Infarction, stroke or any other thrombotic complication [95, 96].

e. Interferon Alpha: Interferon Alpha has demonstrated efficacy in Polycythemia Vera in controlling leukocytosis and thrombocytosis and decreasing the need for phlebotomy. It is often used as first line agent in younger patients and pregnant women. It also prevent the thrombotic complications and in very few studies, has shown reversal of minimal fibrosis in the bone marrow [95, 96, 97].

f. Other Chemotherapeutic Agents: Busalphan and Chlorambucil are the alkylating agents, which were used in PV but increased risk of leukemia had lead to the discontinuation of their use.

Radioactive Phosphorous (32P) is an intravenous agent, which has a good uptake in rapidly multiplying cells. It's uptake in bone, makes it a valuable tool in hematologic disorders. It also has leukomogenic potential, but may take up to seven to ten years, so it should be judiciously used and can be restricted to patients above 75 years [74].

g. Surgery/ Splenectomy: Splenectomy is an option in painful splenomegaly and recurrent thrombosis causing splenic infarction [81, 83, 98, 99].

Phlebotomy is the primary therapy and should be used to decrease the hematocrit to less than 45. The use of Cytoreductive therapy depends on risk stratification of the patients depending on age and other risk factors like history of thrombosis:

Age	Risk Factors	Treatment (Cytoreductive)
Less than 65 years	None	Observation plus low dose Aspirin
Less than 65 years (40-65 years)	Poor tolerance to Phlebotomy. Symptomatic or Progressive splenomegaly.	Aspirin Plus First Line: Interferon. Second line: Hydroxyurea
Age	Risk Factors	Treatment (Cytoreductive)
Greater than 65 Years	Disease progression. Thrombosis like Deep Venous Thrombosis (DVT), Transient Ischemic Attack (TIA), Infarction of any vessels, or stroke. None	or Anagrelide. Aspirin plus Hydroxyurea or Anagrelide

PRIMARY MYELOFIBROSIS (PMF)

The primary myelofibrosis (PMF), also known as chronic idiopathic myelofibrosis (CIMF), agnogenic myeloid metaplasia is a chronic myeloproliferative disorder characterized by clonal hematopoetic stem cell disorder resulting in atypical megakaryocyte hyperplasia and bone marrow fibrosis [100, 101].

Epidemiology

It is usually a disorder of middle and old age, with median age of diagnosis being 67 years [102], with approximately 15-17% of patients being below the age 40-50 years [103]. It is very rarely seen in children [104]. It is the least frequently encountered chronic myeloproliferative disorders with annual incidence of approximately 1.5 cases/100,000 individuals as reported in a study in Minnesota [105].

Etio-pathogenesis

Exact cause for this disease is unknown but a somatic mutation in pluripotent hematopoietic progenitor cells is considered [106, 107], while exposure to thorium oxide, toulene, benzene, ionizing radiation has been suggested in minority of the cases [106, 108, 109].

The primary process of chronic myeloproliferation and atypical hyperplasia [110] leading to abnormal shedding of additional growth factors and cytokines like TGF-b, FGF, EGF, PDGF,VEGF, lysyl oxide and MMP-9 [111, 112]; resulting in non clonal proliferation of fibroblast which in turn leads to bone marrow fibrosis; hallmark of primary myelofibosis (PMF). Bone marrow fibrosis in turn contributes to impaired hematopoiesis, anemia, extramedulary hematopoiesis, splenomegaly.

The substantial increase in bone marrow micro vascular density (MVD) seen in up to 70% of the patients is also considered to be due to increased levels VEGF, bFGF,TGF-b, PDGF. Chromosomal abnormalities are found in approximately 50-60% of the patients with PMF [111, 113-118], with the most common being -20q in 21%, -13q in 20%, abnormal chromosome 1 in 17%, +8 in 15%, +9 in 13%, -7 in 11%, abnormal chromosome 12 in 9% and -5 in 6%.

Most common mutation found in PMF is JAK2; seen in upto 50% of the patient s along with Calreticulin (CALR) and thrombopoetin receptor mutation (MPL) and many others. [119]. Gain in chromosome 9 or 9p that is seen in 13% of cases; is considered to be very important in pathogenesis of PMF, since JAK2 gene abnormality seen in upto 50% of the PMF patients is also located on chromosome 9 [120].

Clinical Presentation

While up to ¼th of the patients with PMF remain asymptomatic, the most common clinical feature is severe fatigue, left upper quadrant discomfort, early satiety, weight loss, fever, bone pain, night sweats [121-126]. Splenomegaly is seen in up to 90% of the patients is secondary to extramedulary hematopoiesis and increased spleenic flow, hepatomegaly seen in upto 40-70% of the patients is result of extramedullary hematopoiesis [122, 125, 126]; that combined with increased splenic flow can result in portal hypertension and subsequent ascites, esophageal/gastric varices, GI bleed and hepatic encephalopathy [127-131].

Extramedullary hematopoiesis can be seen anywhere in the body including lymph nodes, pleura, lung, abdominal cavity, gastrointestinal tract, genitourinary tract, central nervous system and rarely skin; with clinical features depending on body system involved varying from GI bleed, dysuria, effusion, respiratory distress, intracranial hypertension to neurological symptoms, lymphadenopathy and rash [132-144].

Subsequent splenectomy in patients with PMF can result in enlargement in other extramedullary sites resulting in increased symptoms [144, 145]. Patients with PMF are seen with osteoscleosis leading to bone and joint complains in these patients [125], since PMF is hypermetabolic state and can lead to hyperuricemia and gout as well.

Laboratory Finding

Anemia, thrombocytosis and leukocytosis initially then followed by thrombocytopenia and leucopenia as disease progresses, increased alkaline phosphatase, increased LDH, hyperuricemia, increased vitamin B12 [146, 147]. Peripheral smear examination revealing typical tear drop cells, leukoerythroblastic picture also suggest the diagnosis.

Bone Marrow Examination [148-152]

Bone marrow aspiration is difficult and usually yields dry tap in patient with PMF and will ultimately need a biopsy for diagnosis which shows atypical megakaryocyte hyperplasia, thickening and distortion of bone trabeculae. However in early hyper cellular phase of PMF bone marrow may not show such changes. Diagnosis in such cases is made with clinical features, peripheral blood smears, and ruling out PV and CML.

MRI bone marrow can show conversion of fatty marrow to fibrous marrow which is a result of loss of the water content in marrow, and Isotope imaging using iron isotopes can help localize extramedullary sites. JAK2 gene mutation: JAK2 V617F is found in approximately 43 to 63% of the patients with PMF.

Leukemic Transformation (LT)

PMF can transform in to leukemia mostly of myeloid origin. PMF diagnosis usually requires biopsy of the leukemic sites since the blood picture and bone marrow examination will not reveal much due to abnormalities at base line in blood and bone marrow secondary to the advance disease process [153-158].

Major risk factors of LTL

1. Leukemic blasts equal to or more than 3%.
2. Platelet count <100,000/microL

Depending upon the presence of the risk factors risk of LT can go up to 18%. The treatment related poor prognostic factors are erythropoeisis stimulating factors and danazol. LT in patients with PMF is associated with overall poor prognosis. In one study the median survival was around 2.6 months after LT ranging 0 to 24 months, with AML induction therapy inducing remission in zero percent of the patients.

Diagnosis

WHO criteria for the diagnosis of Primary myelofibrosis are as follows: [159-161]

Presence of megakaryocyte proliferation and atypia, usually accompanied by reticulin and or collagen on bone marrow biopsy.
WHO criteria for polycythemia vera (PV), chronic myeloid leukemia (CML), myelodysplastic syndrome (MDS), or other myeloid neoplasm not fulfilled.
Demonstration of a clonal marker (e.g. JAK2 or MPL).
Leukoerythroblastosis.
Palpable splenomegaly.
Anemia.
Increased serum lactate dehydrogenase level.

Diagnosis of post polycythemia vera (PV) and post essential thrombocythemia (ET) myelofibrosis as proposed by international working group for myelofibrosis research and treatment requires presence of 2/2 major and 2/5 minor criteria.

Major Criteria

1. Documentation of a previously diagnosed PV or ET as defined by WHO criteria.

Presence of increased bone marrow fibrosis.

Minor Criteria

1. Progressive anemia or loss of phlebotomy requirement.

Leukoerythroblastic blood picture.

Worsening splenomegaly.

Development of constitutional symptoms (i.e, weight loss, night sweats, unexplained fever).

Increased serum lactate dehydrogenase (post-ET myelofibrosis only).

Differential Diagnosis

Broad differential in this category includes [162-169]: other Myeloid neoplasm: CML, PV, ET, mast cell histiocytosis, myelodysplastic syndrome (MDS), acute meylofibrosis, acute myeloid leukemia (AML FAB M7) and Lymphoid neoplasia: lymphomas, multiple myeloma, hairy cell leukemia. It also includes non hematologic causes of myelofibrosis: renal osteodystrophy, Vitamin D deficiency, Metastatic tumors to bone marrow, infections, connective tissue disorders.

Prognosis [170-179]

Internationally recognized prognostic criteria for PMF are dynamic international prognostic scoring system (DIPSS) and system proposed by international working group for research and treatment of myelofibrosis. This criterion is based on DIPSS and additional 3 risk factors; as described below.

DIPSS criterion
Age >65 years – 1 point

Leukocyte count >25,000/microL – 1 point
Hemoglobin <10 g/dL – 2 points
Circulating blast cells ≥1 percent – 1 point
Presence of constitutional symptoms – 1 point

Patients are divided in risk groups depending on the points as; zero points (low risk), 1 to 2 points (intermediate -1), 3 to 4 points (intermediate -2), 5 to 6 points (high risk).

DIPSS Plus criterion adds 3 additional IPSS independent risk factors, 1. Unfavorable karyoptype (complex karyotype or sole or two abnormalities that include +8, -7/7q-, i(17q), -5/5q-, 12p-, inv[3], or 11q23 rearrangements), 2. Need for transfusion, 3. Thrombocytopenia.

DIPSS low risk score – 0 points
DIPSS intermediate risk-1 score – 1 point
DIPSS intermediate risk-2 score – 2 points
DIPSS high risk score – 3 points
Unfavorable karyotype – 1 point
Platelet count <100,000/microL – 1 point
Need for transfusion– 1 point.

Subsequent classification in risk groups depending on points; zero points (low risk), one point (intermediate -1), two to three points (intermediate -2), four or six points (high risk).

Application of DIPSS plus criterion in one study of 793 PMF patients at Mayo clinic gave a median survival of 15.4, 6.5, 2.9, and 1.3 years for low risk, intermediate-1,intermediate-2 and high risk patients respectively. Another study at Mayo clinic in 299 young patients (<60 y) gave a median survival from time of referral as 20, 14.3, 5.3, and 1.7 years, for Low risk, intermediate-1, intermediate-2 and high risk patients respectively; signifying the importance age in prognosis.

In addition to above factors, various other cytokines, gene mutations are under study to know more about their effects on prognosis in PMF patients.

Treatment

Allogenic hematopoietic cell transplantation (allo-HCT) remains the only curative therapy in patients with PMF, while chemotherapy is being used to provide symptomatic relief to the patients. Asymptomatic and low risk patients with expected median survival of 10-15 years are usually given supportive care. Various treatments are described as below.

1) Allo-HCT

This treatment modality is usually offered to young patients with the development of two or more adverse factors shortly after diagnosis e.g. hemoglobin <10 mg/dl, constitutional symptoms and isolated cytologic abnormalities or blast cell>1% [180, 181]. It has been suggested to offer this mode of treatment to low risk patients who develop adverse prognostic factors; when expected median survival is less than 5 years [182-185].

Common problems with Allo-HCT include limited availability of donors, acute graft versus host disease (GVHD) and graft versus myelofibrosis effects. In one of the large retrospective studies using registry data on 147 PMF patients undergoing allo-HCT with a median age of 53 years (range 20-68 years), 59% of patients had a transplant with matched donor and 31% underwent myeolablative conditioning [186] 54% of the subjects receiving reduced intensity conditioning were of intermediate-2 or high risk according to the IPSS score, and 24 % had previously transformed into acute myeloid leukemia. Of those receiving myeloablative conditioning, the corresponding percentages were 39 and 15 percent, respectively. There was no significant difference in either overall survival or non-relapse mortality between the two conditioning regimens. 90% of the subjects were engrafted. Favorable factors for engraftment include splenectomy prior to HCT, HLA-matched sibling donor, peripheral stem cell use for HCT, and absence of pre-transplant thrombocytopenia.

Four-year overall survival, progression-free survival, and non-relapse mortality were 39, 32, and 39 percent respectively. On multivariate analysis, HLA-identical sibling donor, chronic phase disease, and splenectomy in men had a favorable impact on overall survival.

In another study of 55 patients [187] of PMF with median age of 42 years, five year survival of 83,43 and 31 percent was reported for low, intermediate and high risk patient groups respectively. With overall five year survival of 47 percent, 40 percent of patients were able to achieve complete histo-hematolgic remission. Unfavorable predictors for five year survival were abnormal karyotype pre-transplant, age ≥45 years and absence of grade II to IV acute GVHD. Favorable predictor includes hemoglobin ≥10 gm/dl and absence of osteomyosclerosis [188].

2) Non-myeloablative Allo-HCT

Multiple studies have reported good outcomes especially in a higher median age group. In a retrospective study of 30 patients [189] with primary and secondary myelofibrosis, median age of 65 years (range 60-78 years) and most of the patients received a low intensity conditioning; the three year over all and progression free survival of 45 and 40 percent respectively were reported with day 100 mortality of 13 percent.

In two other series of patients [190, 191] with a median age of 55 (range 32 to 73 years), reported one year treatment related mortality was 16 to 22 percent; with five year overall and event free survival of 62 to 67percent and 46 to 51 percent respectively. A state of complete remission with full donor chimerism and loss of JAK-2 mutation has also been reported using low intensity myeloablation [190-199].

In patients with failed allo-HCT, other options are donor lymphocyte infusion (DLI) and second transplant.

3) Chemotherapies

a. Hydroxurea: The hydroxurea works by inhibiting the deoxynuicleotode synthesis in S phase of cell cycle. Effects of the medication last few days to a week. This is a preferred agent in PMF for the relief of constitutional symptoms, hepatosplenomegaly, thrombocytosis and leukocytosis. This agent is usually started at low doses since many patients with PMF can have cytopenias and doses are then titrated per individual response. Patients with JAK2 V617F mutation seem to have better response than mutation negative patients [200].

b. Busulfan: This is an alkylating agent which have been used in past for symptomatic relief in patients with PMF but high leukomogenic potential and better safety profile of hydroxyurea makes it an unfavorable drug to use in PMF.

c. Ruxolitinib: It is one of the selective JAK2 inhibitors used for patients with severe constitutional symptoms and splenomegaly. It works by blocking JAK/STAT signaling pathway. Its use is associated with significant improvement in splenic size and the constitutional symptoms. As seen in the Comfort trials I and II [201, 202] the dose of medication varies between 5mg twice daily and 20 mg twice daily depending on platelet count of the patient, and the drug needs a slow taper under supervision when needed to stop. Discontinuation [203,

204] of the drug can result in relapse of the disease symptoms, systemic inflammatory response syndrome (SIRS) with hypotension, fever and hypoxia. Ruxolitinib has also been reported to impair T cell immunity by affecting dendritic function [205].

d. Interferon alfa: The drug works by decreasing proliferation of malignant cells and modulating host immune response. Interferon alfa has shown to reduce blood cell counts and improve splenomegaly in approximately 50% of the patients treated. The Pegylated form of interferon alfa requires less frequent dosage and has a slightly better side effect profile [206].

e. Anagrelide: The Anagrelide when used has shown effects on thrmbocytosis and are reversible when discontinued.

f. Thalidomide with prednisone: This combination is thought to work by immunomodulatory effects and combination allows lower dosage of the drug which is better tolerated. Clinical response is seen in approximately 20 to 40% of the patient with improvement in anemia, red cell transfusion independence, cell counts and reduction in spleen size [207, 208]. Side effects includes drowsiness, neuropathy, constipation and neutropenia [209].

g. Lenalinomide: It is an analog to thalidomide and is more potent than thalidomide. It is in use for multiple myeloma and 5q-myelodysplastic syndrome. In patients with symptomatic myelofibrosis it has shown overall response rates of 22% for anemia, 33% splenomegaly, and 50% for thrombocytopenia [210].

h. Pomalidomide: It is a second generation thalidomide under investigation. It also works by its immunomodulatory effects and has shown effects on anemia in phase II trials [211].

i. Etanercept: It is a tumor necrosis factor receptor and its use has been shown improvement in constitutional symptoms in patients [212].

j. Everolimus: It is a mTOR kinase inhibitor currently in investigative trials. Its use in intermediate to high risk PMF and post PV and post ET myeolfibrosis has shown effects with resolution of constitutional symptoms, size of splenomegaly and improvement in pruritis [213].

k. Histone deacetylase inhibitors: this is another class of drugs under clinical trials, and includes Panobinostat and Givinostat. The phase I and II trials have shown some effects on anemia, splenomegaly and constitutional symptoms [214-217].

l. Androgens: This class of drugs is used in patients to improve anemia in combination with steroids.

4) Splenectomy

Patients with symptoms of overt portal hypertension, anemia requiring multiple transfusions, refractory thrombocytopenia and mechanical abdominal discomfort from splenomegaly not responding to Hydroxyurea may be considered for splenectomy [218-220]. Patients with PMF undergoing splenectomy will require detailed assessment for cell counts, sub-clinical DIC and treatment for DIC to avoid increased peri-operative bleeding. Patients of PMF with bleeding problems may require platelet transfusions, cryoprecipitate during surgery based on clotting parameters. Splenectomy carries an operative mortality of approximately 9% [218]. Post splenectomy marked hepatomegaly and increased thrombocytosis can be seen [219, 220], which can be managed by close monitoring and cytoreductive treatment as appropriate [221]. An increased chance of leukemic transformation has also been reported post splenectomy [222].

5) Radiation therapy

Splenic irradiation can be used for symptomatic relief in PMF patients who are poor surgical candidates. Effects are transient and last about 6 months. Severe prolonged pancytopenia can be seen in approximately one fourth of the patients' post-splenic irradiation [223]. Radiation can also be used to alleviate other symptoms like bone pain and other areas of symptomatic extramedullary hematopoiesis.

ESSENTIAL THROMBOCYTHEMIA (ET)

Essential thrombocythemia (ET) is also known as Essential thrombocytosis or primary thrombocytosis is a chronic thrombocythemia is non reactive and does not fit into any other chronic myeloproliferative disorders [224]. It should be a diagnosis of exclusion after the reasons for reactive thrombocytosis and other chronic myeloproliferative disorders have been excluded [225].

Epidemiology

Patients with ET have a near normal life span. There are variable reports of ET incidence. It is as high as approximately 24/100,000 in the United States

[226], however incidence calculated from Olmsted County, Rochester is around 2.5/100,000 population per year [227]. There is a female predominance of 2:1, [228] median age at diagnosis of 60 years with 20% of cases being below the age of 40 [229]. Childhood ET is a very rare condition with estimated incidence of 0.009/100,000 population per year in children under age of 14 years [230, 231]. It can be both sporadic and familial with variations observed in gene mutation [232].

Pathogenesis

Pathogenesis of ET does not involve mutations in thrombopoetin (TPO) and its receptor C-mpl [233]. However autosomal dominant ET is seen to be associated with mutation in TPO, C-mpl or proteins further down the signaling pathway [233]. Megakaryocyte colony growth endogenously is independent of autocrine effects of TPO [234, 235]. Inappropriately normal or high levels of TPO l seen in patients with ET are suspected to be a result of increased stromal production by bone marrow or decreased ligand clearance secondary to decreased C-mpl expression on platelets of patients with ET [236-239]. Whether ET is a clonal disorder is uncertain. Glucose-6-phosphate dehydrogenase based clonal assays suggested clonality of ET and polycythemia vera [240]. Subsequent studies using X linked DNA and transcript analysis demonstrated a variable pattern of lineage involvement which suggested hierarchically different levels of clonal generation [241-243]. Some studies have also demonstrated monoclonal and polyclonal distribution. [244-248].

Clinical Picture

At the time of diagnosis upto one third patients remain clinically asymptomatic. The vasomotor symptoms such as, headache, dizziness, lightheadedness, acral paresthesia, livedo reticularis, erythromelalgia, transient visual disturbances (ophthalmic migraine, amaurosis fugax, scintillating scotomata) are seen in up to 40% of patients. [249, 250]. Thrombotic and hemorrhagic symptoms occur in 9-22% and 3-37% respectively [251-256] with major bleeding or thrombotic episodes in 7 and 4 percent respectively. The thrombotic symptoms can include transient ischemic attack (TIA), renal artery and vein thrombosis, coronary artery ischemia, deep venous thrombosis

(DVT), pulmonary embolism (PE), hepatic or portal vein thrombosis and digital ischemia.

Rate of thrombotic and hemorrhagic episodes after diagnosis over a median follow up of 3 to 7 years was found to be 7 − 17% and 8 to 14% respectively [251-253, 255, 256]. In one study the factors of thrombosis includes age ≥60 years, previous history of thrombosis, WBC count >11,000, cardiovascular risk factors (tobacco, HTN, DM) and presence of JAK2 V617F mutation. The study also described the rate of fatal and non fatal thrombosis of 1.9 per 100 patients over median follow up of 6.2 years [257].

Females using oral contraceptive were found to have a threefold increase in venous thrombosis (23 versus 7 percent) and a 5 fold increase in splanchnic thrombosis (15 versus 3 percent). Estrogen containing hormone replacement was not associated with increased risk of arterial or venous thrombosis [258].

ET can transform to PV, AML, PMF in 2.7, 1.4 and 4 % of cases respectively over a median follow up of 9.2 years [259]. Other retrospectives studies reported AML incidence ranging from 0.6 to 5 % over three to seven years follow up [250, 252, 253, 260, 261]. Transformation of ET to myelofibrosis with myeloid metaplasia (MMM) has also been reported. The effects of specific ET treatment on risk for MMM are unclear. The prognosis and treatment of post ET MMM compared to de novo MMM is also conjectured. Spontaneous abortion rate is approximately 43% with 36% occurring in first trimester. Other complications include premature delivery 8%, still birth 5%, preeclampsia 4% and fetal growth retardation 4% [262, 263]. One study noted a reduced rate of miscarriages with aspirin with or without heparin [264], but this study received criticism due to selection bias. On physical exam splenomegaly can be found in 24-48% of patients with ET however hepatomegaly and lymphadenopathy are uncommon [265].

Diagnosis

There are two major diagnostic criteria in use for the diagnosis of ET. One is Polycythemia Vera Study Group (PVSG) which is considered the gold standard in diagnosis and other is WHO criteria. There are minor differences in between the two. The most important consideration is excluding other possible causes of thrombocythemia [266]

Polycythemia Vera Study Group (PVSG) Criteria

a)   Platelet count >450,000/microlitre (previously >600,000/microlitre),
b)   Megakaryocytic hyperplasia on bone marrow biopsy and aspiration,
c)   Absence of BCR/ABL on cytogenetic molecular studies and Philadelphia chromosome on karyotype,
d)   Absence of other causes of reactive thrombocytosis.
e)   Normal ferritn levels, normal Mean Corpuscular Volume (MCV) and normal Red Cell Mass levels except in patients with hematocrit (Hct %) less than 40.

Two common mutations seen in patients with ET include JAk2617V>F seen in 50 to 64% of cases [248, 267-270] and clacinuerin mutation seen in 15-25% of cases [269-272]. JAK2617V>F has been observed with high hemoglobin levels, increased total WBC count, increased transformation to PV and increased thrombosis [273-278]. Calcinuerin is seen in younger, male patients and is associated with lower incidence of thrombosis [269-271, 279].

Differential Diagnosis

1)   Reactive thrombocytosis caused by non malignant hematologic conditions, other malignancies, infections, drugs, tissue trauma, exercise, allergies and asplenia whether functional or surgical.
2)   CML is characterized by positive BCR/ABL and Philadelphia chromosome.
3)   PV is characterized by the presence of JAK2 mutation and increased red cell mass.
4)   PMF can be confused with ET in early stages of disease on bone marrow biopsy. The megarkaryocyte proliferation, atypia, degree of bone marrow fibrosis leukoerythroblastic picture on peripheral blood and splenomegaly can help differentiate it from ET.
5)   Myelodysplastic syndrome (MDS) is usually associated with thrombocytopenia; however thrombocytosis can be associated with certain deletion like -5q, 3q21 q26 and refractory anemia with ringed sideroblasts.

Prognosis and Survival

An international study of 891 patients with ET diagnosed with WHO criteria led to international prognostic system for ET (IPSET) which was later validated in to two cohorts [280]. Median survival of patients with ET was different on following factors; age >60 (2 points), WBC count >11,000 (1 point), prior history of thrombosis (1 point). Based on these 3 survival groups were assembled. Median survival for low risk (total points zero) was not reached, for intermediate risk (total points 1 or 2) was 24.5 years, and for high risk (total points >2) was 13.8 years.

Multivariate analysis of 155 deaths among 605 ET patients followed for 7 years suggested that low hemoglobin < 12 mg/dl was an additional factor for survival [281].

As predicted from IPSET, 10 year thrombosis free interval for patient with low, intermediate and high risk patient was approximately 89, 84, and 69 percent respectively [282]. Independent risk factors as predicted from cohort of 891 patients are age >60 years (HR 1.5; 1 point), history of thrombosis (HR 1.9; 2 points), presence of cardiovascular risk factors (diabetes, hypertension, smoking, HR 1.6; 1 point), and presence of the JAK2 V617F mutation (HR 2.0; 2 points).

Based on these factors, three risk groups were compiled. 1) low risk for thrombosis (total score zero or 1) − 1.03%/year risk of thrombosis, 2) intermediate risk (total score 2) − 2.35 percent/year, 3) high risk (total score >2) − 3.56 percent/year.

Overall bleeding risk in ET patients over the course of disease is predicted to be low [283] and use of low dose aspirin (40-100 mg /day) does not seem to increase the risk of bleeding unless the patient has platelet count <1000,000, prior history of bleed or acquired von Willebrand factor deficiency [284, 285]. In a study of 605 patients followed for 7 years, leukemic transformation (LT) was seen in 20 patients (3.3%). Risk factors for LT are [281] low hemoglobin level (<12 g/dL in females, <13.5 in males), Platelet count ≥1,000,000/microL and increased age.

TREATMENT

Most patient with ET are asymptomatic and do not require any treatment. Treatment is only indicated in patient who is high risk of thrombosis such as age > 60 and history of thrombosis [82]. Vasomotor symptoms are common in

ET and can be easily managed with aspirin alone with doses from 40 to 100 mg/day [286, 287]. Aspirin is also indicated in patient with other risk factors such as cardiac disease.

Low risk patient (age less than 60, no history of prior thrombosis) with an elevated platelet count >1 million should be screened for acquired von Willebrand factor deficiency by ristocetin cofactor assay. Aspirin up to 100 mg/day should be given when ristocetin cofactor activity exceeds 30 percent. Modification of other risk factors such as obesity, smoking, hypertension, hyperlipidemia should also be considered to further reduce the risk of thrombosis.

Cytoreductive therapy is considered only in high risk patients. One treatment to consider is hydroxyurea. This medication works by inhibiting enzyme ribonucleotide reductase in DNA synthesis; leading to reduction in platelet count. Hydroxyurea is the preferred medication in high risk ET patients. Medication effects can be seen in 4-5 days, with a rising MCV indicates effectiveness of the drug. Goal is to keep the platelet level from 100,000 to 400,000 mg/L. Common side effects associated with hydroxyurea are mouth ulcers, skin pigmentation, skin rash and nail changes [288]. Less frequently patients can develop diarrhea, alopecia, or leg ulcers [289]. Abnormal liver function tests and fever can be rare side effects of hydroxyurea. Pregnant, or breast feeding women or women of child bearing age should not take this medication. Anemia or leucopenia can be seen in patients taking hydroxyurea so complete blood count and liver function tests are appropriate for monitoring the potential side effects of hydroxyurea.

The anagrelide comes from the imidazoquinazoline group of drugs which decreases platelet production by affecting proliferation and maturation. At higher doses anagrelide inhibits platelet aggregation via anti cyclic AMP phosphodiesterase pathway [290-292]. Common side effects associated with this medication includes headache, palpitation, fluid retention, tachycardia and diarrhea [293]. Anagrelide has also been associated with development of idiopathic cardiomyopathy [294]. Anagrelide may cause high output heart failure which warrants the cautious use of this medication in cardiac patients and the elderly [295].

Based on data from the randomized trial, UK research council primary thrombocythemia study 1, hydroxyurea with aspirin has fewer side effects compared to anagrelide with aspirin when used in high risk ET patients. A lower incidence of arterial thrombosis, venous thrombosis and progression to myelofibrosis was noted in this study [296].

Interferon alpha works by direct myelosuppressive effects leading to decrease in platelet count, however clonal proliferation continues so rebound growth in platelet can be seen after interferon is stopped [297]. Interferon alpha does not cross the placenta and is not considered teratogenic. Pegylated interferon is a more convenient form of interferon that has similar efficacy.

Pipobroman is an alkylating agent widely used in Europe but not available in US.

Platephoresis is a transient measure to decrease the platelet count. It can be helpful in acute, serious, thrombotic or hemorrhagic complications [298, 299]. Ultimately all such patients need a myelosuppressive treatment to keep platelet count below 400,000 mg/L.

REFERENCES

[1]   Champlin RE, Golde DW. Chronic myelogenous leukemia: recent advances. *Blood* 1985;65:1039-1047.

[2]   Bennett, J.H. (1845) Case of hypertrophy of the spleen and liver in which death took place from suppuration of the blood. *Edinburgh Medical and Surgical Journal,* 64, 413±423.

[3]   Virchow R. Gesammelte Abhandlungen zur wissenschaftlichen Medizin. Hamm CGrotesche. *Buchdlung 1862*;192.

[4]   Virchow R. Zur pathologischen Physiologie des Blutes. *Arch Pathol Anat Physiol Klin Med* 1849;2:592.

[5]   Neumann E. Uber myeogene Leukmie. *Berl Klin Wochenschr* 1878;15:116.

[6]   Nowell PC, Hungerford DA. A minutes chromosome in human granulocytic leukemia. *Science* 1960;132:1497.

[7]   Rowley JD. A new consistent chromosomal abnormality in chronic myelogenous leukaemia identified by quinacrine fluorescence and Giemsa staining. *Nature* 1973;243:290-293.

[8]   Kurzrock R, Gutterman JU, Talpz M. The molecular genetics of Philadelphia chromosome positive leukemias. *N Engl J Med* 1988;319:990-998

[9]   Heisterkamp N, Knoppel E, Groffen J. The first BCR gene intron contains breakpoints in the Philadelphia chromosome positive leukemia. *Nucleic Acids Res* 1988;16:10069-10081.

[10]   Timmons MS, Witte ON. Structural characterization of the BCR gene product. *Oncogene* 1989;4:559-567.

[11] Chissoe SL, Bodenteich A, Wang YF, et al. Sequence and analysis of the human ABL gene, the BCR gene, and regions involved in the Philadelphia chromosomal translocations. *Genomics* 1995;27:67-82.

[12] Wada HM, Mizutani S, Nishimura J, et al. Establishment and molecular characterization of a novel leukemic cell line with Philadelphia chromosome expressing p230 BCR/ABL fusion protein. *Cancer Res* 1995;55:3192-3196.

[13] Guo JQ, Wang JY, Arlinghaus RB. Detection of BCR-ABL proteins in blood cells of beginning phase of chronic myelogenous leukemia patients. *Cancer Res* 1991;51:3048-3051.

[14] Gorska-Flipot I, Norman C, Addy L, et al. Molecular pathology of chronic myelogenous leukemia. *Tumour Biol* 1990;11[Suppl 1]:25-43.

[15] Moloney WC. Natural history of chronic granulocytic leukaemia. *Clin Haematol* 1977;6:41-53.

[16] Rowe JM, Lichtman MA. Hyperleukocytosis and leukostasis: common features of childhood chronic myelogenous leukemia. *Blood* 1984;63:1230-1234.

[17] Kamada N, Uchino H. Chronologic sequence in appearance of clinical and laboratory findings characteristic of chronic myelocytic leukemia. *Blood* 1978;51:843-850.

[18] Melo JV. The diversity of BCR-ABL fusion proteins and their relationship to leukemia phenotype. *Blood* 1996;88:2375-2384.

[19] Tuszynski A, Dhut S, Toung BD, et al. Detection and significance of bcr-abl mRNA transcripts and fusion proteins in Philadelphia positive adult acute lymphoblastic leukemia. *Leukemia* 1993;7:1504-1508.

[20] Secker-Walker LM, Cooke HM, Browett PJ, et al. Variable Philadelphia breakpoints and potential lineage restriction of bcr rearrangement in acute lymphoblastic leukemia. *Blood* 1988;72:784-791.

[21] Radich JP, Kopecky KJ, Boldt DH, et al. Detection of BCR-ABL fusion genes in adult acute lymphoblastic leukemia by polymerase chain reaction. *Leukemia* 1994;8:1688-1695

[22] Kantarjian HM, Talpaz M, Dhingra K, et al. Significance of the p210 versus the p190 molecular abnormalities in adults with Philadelphia chromosome positive acute leukemia. *Blood* 1991;78:2411-2418.

[23] Martiat P, Mecucci C, Nizet Y, et al. P190 BCR/ABL transcript in case of Philadelphia chromosome positive multiple myeloma. *Leukemia* 1990;4:751-754. P.2255

[24] Mitani K, Sato Y, Tojo A, et al. Philadelphia chromosome positive B cell type malignant lymphoma expressing an aberrant 190kd bcr-abl protein. *Br J Haematol* 1990;76:221-224.

[25] Bedi A, Barber JP, Bedi GC, el-Deiry WS, Sidransky D, Vala MS, Akhtar AJ, Hilton J, Jones RJ. BCR-ABL-mediated inhibition of apoptosis with delay of G2/M transition after DNA damage: a mechanism of resistance to multiple anticancer agents. *Blood.* 1995 Aug 1;86(3):1148–1158.

[26] Thompson DS, Stainsby D. The clinical and haematological features of chronic granulocytic leukaemia in the chronic phase. In: Shaw M, editor. *Chronic Granulocytic Leukaemia.* New York: Praeger; 1982. pp137–188.

[27] Cortes JE, Talpaz M, Kantarjian H. Chronic myelogenous leukemia: a review. *Am J Med.* 1996;100:555-570.

[28] Goldman JM. Chronic myeloid leukemia. *Curr Opin Hematol.* 1997;4:277-285.

[29] Inbal A. A retrospective study of patients with chronic myeloid leukemia diagnosed and treated at the Chaim Sheba Medical Center during the years 1966-76. *Isr J Med Sci* 1978;14:1259-1264.

[30] Kardinal CG, Bateman JR, Weinter J. Chronic granulocytic leukemia: review of 536 cases. *Arch Intern Med* 1976;136:305-313.

[31] Cortes J, O'Dwyer ME. Clonal evolution in chronic myelogenous leukemia. *Hematol Oncol Clin North Am.* 2004;18:671–84. doi: 10.1016/j.hoc.2004.03.012

[32] Karyotype abnormalities and their clinical significance in blast crisis of chronic myeloid leukemia. Griesshammer M, Heinze B, Bangerter M, Heimpel H, Fliedner TM. *J Mol Med* (Berl). 1997 Nov-Dec;75(11-12):836-8.

[33] Schilling RF, Crowley JJ. Prognostic signs in chronic myelocytic leukemia. *Am J Hematol* 1979;7:1-10.

[34] Hyun BH, Gulati GL, Ashton JK. Myeloproliferative disorders: classification and diagnostic features with special emphasis on chronic myelogenous leukemia and agnogenic myeloid metaplasia. *Clin Lab Med* 1990;10:825-838.

[35] Spiers AS. Chronic granulocytic leukemia. *Med Clin North Am* 1984;68:713-727

[36] Lorand-Metze I, Vassalo J, Souza CA. Histological and cytological heterozygosity of bone marrow in Philadelphia positive chronic myelogenous leukemia at diagnosis. *Br J Haematol* 1987;67:45-49.

[37] Mitelman F. The cytogenetic scenario of chronic myeloid leukemia. *Leuk Lymphoma* 1993;11[Suppl 1]:11-15.

[38] T-cell cytogenetics in chronic granulocytic leukaemia. Kearney L, Orchard KH, Hibbin J, Goldman JM. *Lancet.* 1982 Apr 10;1(8276):858

[39] T lymphocytes lack rearrangement of the bcr gene in Philadelphia chromosome- Positive chronic myeloid leukemia. Bartram CR, Raghavachar A, Anger B, Stain C, Bettelheim P. *Blood.* 1987 Jun;69(6):1682-5.

[40] The application of fluorescent in situ hybridization to detect Mbcr/abl fusion in variant Ph Chromosomes in CML. Dewald GW, Schad CR, Christensen ER, Tiede AL, Zinsmeister AR, Spurbeck JL, Thibodeau SN, Jalal SM. *Cancer Genet Cytogenet.* 1993 Nov;71(1):7-14.

[41] Bolufer P, Sanz GF, Barragán E, Sanz MA, Cervera J, Lerma E, Senent L, Moreno I, Planelles. Haematologica. *Rapid quantitative detection of BCR-ABL transcripts in chronic myeloid leukemia patients by real-time reverse transcriptase polymerase-chain reaction using fluorescently labeled probes* 2000 Dec;85(12):1248-54.

[42] Imatinib mesylate: clinical results in Philadelphia chromosome-positive leukemias. Kantarjian HM, Talpaz M. *Semin Oncol.* 2001 Oct;28(5 Suppl 17):9-18.

[43] O'Brien SG, Guilhot F, Larson RA, et al. Imatinib compared with interferon and low-dose cytarabine for newly diagnosed chronic-phase chronic myeloid leukemia. *N Engl J Med* 2003; 348:994.

[44] Druker BJ, Guilhot F, O'Brien SG, et al. Five-year follow-up of patients receiving imatinib for chronic myeloid leukemia. *N Engl J Med* 2006; 355:2408.

[45] Chronic myeloid leukemia: an update of concepts and management recommendations of European LeukemiaNet. Baccarani M, Cortes J, Pane F, Niederwieser D, Saglio G, Apperley J, Cervantes F, Deininger M, Gratwohl A, Guilhot F, Hochhaus A, Horowitz M, Hughes T,Kantarjian H, Larson R, Radich J, Simonsson B, Silver RT, Goldman J, Hehlmann R; European LeukemiaNet. *J Clin Oncol.* 2009 Dec 10;27(35):6041-51.

[46] Talpaz M,Kantarjian HM,McCredie KB,Keating MJ,Trujillo J,Gutterman J. Clinical investigation of human alpha interferon in chronic myelogenous leukemia. *Blood.* 1987; 69: 1280–1288.

[47] Kantarjian H,O'Brien S,Cortes J, et al. Complete cytogenetic and molecular responses to interferon-α-based therapy for chronic

myelogenous leukemia are associated with excellent long-term prognosis. *Cancer.* 2003; 97: 1033–1041.

[48]   Talpaz M, Shah N, Kantarjian H, et al. Dasatinib in imatinib-resistant Philadelphia-chromosome positive leukemias. *N Engl J Med* 2006;354:2531–2541.

[49]   Kantarjian H, Sawyers C, Hochhaus A, et al: Hematologic and cytogenetic responses to imatinib mesylate in chronic myelogenous leukemia. *N Engl J Med* 346:645-652, 2002.

[50]   Bruemmendorf TH, Cervantes F, Kim D, et al: Bosutinib is safe and active in patients (pts) with chronic phase (CP) chronic myeloid leukemia (CML) with resistance or intolerance to imatinib and other tyrosine kinase inhibitors. *J Clin Oncol* 26:372s, 2008 (suppl; abstr 7001)

[51]   Hochhaus A, Kantarjian HM, Baccarani M, et al: Dasatinib induces notable hematologic and cytogenetic responses in chronic-phase chronic myeloid leukemia after failure of imatinib therapy. *Blood* 109:2303-2309, 2007

[52]   Kantarjian HM, Giles F, Gattermann N, et al: Nilotinib (formerly AMN107), a highly selective BCR-ABL tyrosine kinase inhibitor, is effective in patients with Philadelphia chromosome-positive chronic myelogenous leukemia in chronic phase following imatinib resistance and intolerance. *Blood* 110:3540-3546,2007

[53]   Quintas-Cardama A, Kantarjian H, Jones D, et al: Dasatinib (BMS-354825) is active in Philadelphia chromosome-positive chronic myelogenous leukemia after imatinib and nilotinib (AMN107) therapy failure. *Blood* 109:497-499, 2007

[54]   Disappearance of Ph1-positive cells in four patients with chronic granulocytic leukemia after chemotherapy, irradiation and marrow transplantation from an identical twin. Fefer A, Cheever MA, Thomas ED, Boyd C, Ramberg R, Glucksberg H, Buckner CD, Storb R. *N Engl J Med.* 1979 Feb 15;300(7):333-7.

[55]   Galimberti M, Polchi P, Lucarelli G, et al. Allogeneic marrow transplantation in patients with chronic myeloid leukemia in chronic phase following preparation with busulfan and cyclophosphamide. *Bone Marrow Transplant* 1994;13:197-201.

[56]   Brodsky I, Biggs JC, Szer J, et al. Treatment of chronic myelogenous leukemia with allogeneic bone marrow transplantation after preparation with busulfan and cyclophosphamide (BuCy2): an update. *Semin Oncol* 1993;20:27-32.

[57] Santos GW. Busulfan and cyclophosphamide versus cyclophosphamide and total body irradiation for marrow transplantation in chronic myelogenous leukemia: a review. *Leuk Lymphoma* 1993;11:201-204.

[58] Froberg MK, Brunning RD, Dorion P, et al. Demonstration of clonality in neutrophils using FISH in a case of chronic neutrophilic leukemia. *Leukemia.* 1998;12:623-626.

[59] Yanagiasawa K, Ohminami H, Sata M, et al. Neoplastic involvement of granulocytic lineage, not granulocytic-monocytic, monocytic or erythrocytic lineage, in a patient with chronic neutrophilic leukemia. *Am J Hematol.* 1998;57:221-224.

[60] Di Donata C, Croci G, Lazzari S, et al Chronic neutrophilic leukemia: description of a new case with karyotypic abnormalities. *Am J Clin Pathol.* 1986;85:369-371

[61] Chusid MJ, Dale DC, West BC, Wolff SM. The hypereosinophilic syndrome: analysis of fourteen cases with review of the literature. *Medicine.* 1975;54:1-27.

[62] Bain BJ. Eosinophilic leukaemias and the idiopathic hypereosinophilic syndrome. *Br J Haematol.* 1996;95:2-9

[63] Chronic eosinophilic leukemia with FIP1L1-PDGFRA transcripts after occupational and therapeutic exposure to radiation. Balatzenko G, Stoyanov N, Bekrieva E, Guenova M. Hematol Rep. 2011 Aug 31;3(2):e17. doi: 10.4081/hr.2011.e17. Epub 2011 Oct 11

[64] Groupe Francais de Cytogenetique Hematologique. Chronic myelomonocytic leukemia: single entity or heterogeneous disorder? A prospective multicenter study of 100 patients. *Cancer Genet Cytogenet. 1991*;55:57-65

[65] Groupe Francais de Cytogenetique Hematologique. Chronic myelomonocytic leukemia: single entity or heterogeneous disorder? A prospective multicenter study of 100 patients. *Cancer Genet Cytogenet.*1991;55:57-65

[66] Talarico LD. Myeloproliferative disorders: a practical review. *Patient Care* 1998; 30:37–57.

[67] Berlin NI. Diagnosis and classification of the polycythemias. *Semin Hematol. Oct* 1975;12(4):339-51.

[68] McMullin MF. Int J Lab Hematol. *The classification and diagnosis of erythrocytosis.* 2008 Dec;30(6):447-59.. Epub 2008 Sep 23. Review.

[69] Streiff MB, Smith B, Spivak JL. The diagnosis and management of polycythemia vera in the era since the Polycythemia Vera Study Group:

a survey of American Society of Hematology members' practice patterns. *Blood. Feb* 15 2002;99(4):1144-9

[70]   James C, Ugo V, Le Couedic JP, et al. A unique clonal JAK2 mutation leading to constitutive signalling causes polycythaemia vera. *Nature. Apr* 28 2005;434(7037):1144-8

[71]   Kralovics R, Teo SS, Buser AS, et al. Altered gene expression in myeloproliferative disorders correlates with activation of signaling by the V617F mutation of Jak2. *Blood.* Nov 15 2005;106(10):3374-6.

[72]   Myeloproliferative disorders. Levine RL, Gilliland DG. Blood. 2008 Sep 15;112(6):2190-8. doi: 10.1182/blood-2008-03-077966. Review.

[73]   Hoffman R, Benz EJ Jr, Shattil SJ, et al. *Hematology: Basic Principles and Practice.* 3rd ed. New York, NY: Churchill Livingstone; 2000:1106-1155, 1172-1205.

[74]   Bilgrami S, Greenbeg BR. Polycythemia rubra vera. *Semin Oncol* 1995; 22:307–326.

[75]   Saini KS, Patnaik MM, Tefferi A (2010). "Polycythemia vera-associated pruritus and its management". *Eur J Clin Invest* 40 (9): 828–34

[76]   van Genderen P, Michiels J (1997). "Erythromelalgia: a pathognomonic microvascular thrombotic complication in essential thrombocythemia and polycythemia vera". *Semin Thromb Hemost* 23 (4): 357–63.

[77]   Pathophysiology of thrombosis in myeloproliferative neoplasms. Landolfi R, Di Gennaro L. *Haematologica.* 2011 Feb;96(2):183-6. doi: 0.3324/haematol.2010.038299

[78]   Thrombosis and bleeding in polycythemia vera and essential thrombocythemia: pathogenetic mechanisms and prevention. Landolfi R, Cipriani MC, Novarese L. *Best Pract Res Clin Haematol.* 2006;19(3):617-33. Review.

[79]   Myeloproliferative neoplasms in Budd-Chiari syndrome and portal vein thrombosis: a meta-analysis. Smalberg JH, Arends LR, Valla DC, Kiladjian JJ, Janssen HL, Leebeek FW. *Blood.* 2012 Dec 13;120(25):4921-8.

[80]   Polycythemia vera: the natural history of 1213 patients followed for 20 years. Gruppo Italiano Studio Policitemia. *Ann Intern Med.* 1995 Nov 1;123(9):656-64.

[81]   *Polycythemia Vera and the Myeloproliferative Disorders.* Edited by Louis R. Wasserman, Paul D. Berk, and Nathaniel I. Berlin. 361 pp., illustrated. Philadelphia, W.B. Saunders, 1995

[82]   Minot G, Buckman TE. Erythremia (polycythemia vera): the development of anemia; the relation to leukemia; consideration of the

basal metabolism, blood formation and destruction and fragility of the red cells. *Am J Med Sci.* 1923;166:469-488

[83]   Lawrence JH, Berlin NI, Huff RL. The nature and treatment of polycythemia. *Medicine.* 1953;32:323-388.

[84]   Osgood EE. *Contrasting incidence of acute monocytic and granulocytic leukemias in P32-treated patients with polycythemia vera and chronic lymphocytic leukemia*

[85]   Vardiman JW, Thiele J, Arber DA, et al. The 2008 Revision of the World Health Organization (WHO) classification of myeloid neoplasms and acute leukemia: rationale and important changes [published online ahead of print April 8, 2009]. *Blood* 2009; 114:937–951.

[86]   Diagnostic criteria of the myeloproliferative disorders (MPD): essential thrombocythaemia, polycythaemia veraand chronic megakaryocytic granulocytic metaplasia. Michiels JJ. *Neth J Med.* 1997 Aug;51(2):57-64

[87]   Kilbridge TM, Fried W, Heller P. The mechanism by which plethora suppresses erythropoiesis. *Blood.* 1969;33:104-113.

[88]   Cazzola M, Guarnone R, Cerani P, et al. Red blood cell precursor mass as an independent determinant of serum erythropoietin level. *Blood.*1998;91:2139-2145.

[89]   Influence of the assays of endogenous colony formation and serum erythropoietin on the diagnosis of polycythemia vera and essential thrombocythemia. Mossuz P; Groupe d'Etudes Multicentriques des Syndrome MyéloProlifératifs (GEMSMP). *Semin Thromb Hemost.* 2006 Apr;32(3):246-50. Review.

[90]   Stephens DJ, Kaltreider N. The therapeutic use of venesection in polycythemia. *Ann Intern Med.* 1937;10:1565-1581.

[91]   Kaboth U, Rumpf KW, Lipp T, et al. Treatment of polycythemia vera by isovolemic large-volume erythrocytapheresis. *Klin Wochenschr.* 1990;68:18-25

[92]   Weinfeld A, Swolin B, Westin J. Acute leukaemia after hydroxyurea therapy in polycythaemia vera and allied disorders: prospective study of efficacy and leukaemogenicity with therapeutic implications. Eur *J Haematol.* Mar 1994;52(3):134-9.

[93]   Fruchtman SM, Mack K, Kaplan ME, et al. From efficacy to safety: a Polycythemia Vera Study Group report on hydroxyurea in patients with polycythemia vera. *Semin Hematol.* Jan 1997;34(1):17-23.

[94]   Anagrelide Study Group. Anagrelide, a therapy for thrombocythemic states: experience in 577 patients. *Am J Med. Jan* 1992;92(1):69-76.

[95]   Passamonti F. How to manage polycythemia vera. *Leukemia.* Dec 9 2011

[96]   Landolfi R, Marchioli R, Kutti J, et al. Efficacy and safety of low-dose aspirin in polycythemia vera. *N Engl J Med.* Jan 8 2004;350(2):114-24.

[97]   Cimino R, Rametta V, Matera C, et al. Recombinant interferon alpha-2b in the treatment of polycythemia vera. *Am J Hematol.* Nov 1993;44(3):155-7.

[98]   Symptomatic splenomegaly in polycythemia vera: a review of the indications for splenectomy and perioperative considerations. Logan MS, Watson CM, Nottingham JM. *Am Surg.* 2009 May;75(5):363-8

[99]   How I treat patients with polycythemia vera. Finazzi G, Barbui T. *Blood.* 2007 Jun 15;109(12):5104-11. Epub 2007 Jan 30. Review.

[100] Mesa RA, Verstovsek S, Cervantes F, et al. Primary myelofibrosis (PMF), post polycythemia vera myelofibrosis (post-PV MF), post essential thrombocythemia myelofibrosis (post-ET MF), blast phase PMF (PMF-BP): Consensus on terminology by the international working group for myelofibrosis research and treatment (IWG-MRT). *Leuk Res* 2007; 31:737.

[101] Tefferi A. Myelofibrosis with myeloid metaplasia. *N Engl J Med* 2000; 342:1255.

[102] Mesa RA, Silverstein MN, Jacobsen SJ, et al. Population-based incidence and survival figures in essential thrombocythemia and agnogenic myeloid metaplasia: an Olmsted County Study, 1976-1995. *Am J Hematol* 1999; 61:10.

[103] Visani G, Finelli C, Castelli U, et al. Myelofibrosis with myeloid metaplasia: clinical and haematological parameters predicting survival in a series of 133 patients. *Br J Haematol* 1990; 75:4.

[104] DeLario MR, Sheehan AM, Ataya R, et al. Clinical, histopathologic, and genetic features of pediatric primary myelofibrosis--an entity different from adults. *Am J Hematol* 2012; 87:461.

[105] Mesa RA, Silverstein MN, Jacobsen SJ, et al. Population-based incidence and survival figures in essential thrombocythemia and agnogenic myeloid metaplasia: an Olmsted County Study, 1976-1995. *Am J Hematol* 1999; 61:10.

[106] Smith RE, Chelmowski MK, Szabo EJ. Myelofibrosis: a review of clinical and pathologic features and treatment. *Crit Rev Oncol Hematol* 1990; 10:305.

[107] Campbell PJ, Green AR. The myeloproliferative disorders. *N Engl J Med* 2006; 355:2452.

[108] Bosch X, Campistol JM, Montoliu J, et al. Toluene-associated myelofibrosis. *Blut* 1989; 58:219.

[109] Bosch X, Campistol JM, Montoliu J, Revert L. Myelofibrosis and focal segmental glomerulosclerosis associated with toluene poisoning. *Hum Toxicol* 1988; 7:357.

[110] Ciurea SO, Merchant D, Mahmud N, et al. Pivotal contributions of megakaryocytes to the biology of idiopathic myelofibrosis. *Blood* 2007; 110:986.

[111] Tefferi A. Pathogenesis of myelofibrosis with myeloid metaplasia. *J Clin Oncol* 2005; 23:8520.

[112] Kimura A, Katoh O, Kuramoto A. Effects of platelet derived growth factor, epidermal growth factor and transforming growth factor-beta on the growth of human marrow fibroblasts. *Br J Haematol* 1988; 69:9.

[113] Dupriez B, Morel P, Demory JL, et al. Prognostic factors in agnogenic myeloid metaplasia: a report on 195 cases with a new scoring system. *Blood* 1996; 88:1013.

[114] Reilly JT, Snowden JA, Spearing RL, et al. Cytogenetic abnormalities and their prognostic significance in idiopathic myelofibrosis: a study of 106 cases. *Br J Haematol* 1997; 98:96.

[115] Sinclair EJ, Forrest EC, Reilly JT, et al. Fluorescence in situ hybridization analysis of 25 cases of idiopathic myelofibrosis and two cases of secondary myelofibrosis: monoallelic loss of RB1, D13S319 and D13S25 loci associated with cytogenetic deletion and translocation involving 13q14. *Br J Haematol* 2001; 113:365.

[116] Tefferi A, Mesa RA, Schroeder G, et al. Cytogenetic findings and their clinical relevance in myelofibrosis with myeloid metaplasia. *Br J Haematol* 2001; 113:763.

[117] Tefferi A, Dingli D, Li CY, Dewald GW. Prognostic diversity among cytogenetic abnormalities in myelofibrosis with myeloid metaplasia. *Cancer* 2005; 104:1656.

[118] Strasser-Weippl K, Steurer M, Kees M, et al. Prognostic relevance of cytogenetics determined by fluorescent in situ hybridization in patients having myelofibrosis with myeloid metaplasia. *Cancer* 2006; 107:2801.

[119] Pikman Y, Lee BH, Mercher T, et al. MPLW515L is a novel somatic activating mutation in myelofibrosis with myeloid metaplasia. *PLoS Med* 2006; 3:e270.

[120] Al-Assar O, Ul-Hassan A, Brown R, et al. Gains on 9p are common genomic aberrations in idiopathic myelofibrosis: a comparative genomic hybridization study. *Br J Haematol* 2005; 129:66.

[121] Mesa RA, Silverstein MN, Jacobsen SJ, et al. Population-based incidence and survival figures in essential thrombocythemia and agnogenic myeloid metaplasia: an Olmsted County Study, 1976-1995. *Am J Hematol* 1999; 61:10.

[122] Visani G, Finelli C, Castelli U, et al. Myelofibrosis with myeloid metaplasia: clinical and haematological parameters predicting survival in a series of 133 patients. *Br J Haematol* 1990; 75:4.

[123] Smith RE, Chelmowski MK, Szabo EJ. Myelofibrosis: a review of clinical and pathologic features and treatment. *Crit Rev Oncol Hematol* 1990; 10:305.

[124] Cervantes F, Pereira A, Esteve J, et al. Identification of 'short-lived' and 'long-lived' patients at presentation of idiopathic myelofibrosis. *Br J Haematol* 1997; 97:635.

[125] Silverstein MN. *Agnogenic myeloid metaplasia,* Publishing Sciences Group, Acton, MA 1975.

[126] Varki A, Lottenberg R, Griffith R, Reinhard E. The syndrome of idiopathic myelofibrosis. A clinicopathologic review with emphasis on the prognostic variables predicting survival. *Medicine* (Baltimore) 1983; 62:353.

[127] García-Manero G, Schuster SJ, Patrick H, Martinez J. Pulmonary hypertension in patients with myelofibrosis secondary to myeloproliferative diseases. *Am J Hematol* 1999; 60:130.

[128] Dingli D, Utz JP, Krowka MJ, et al. Unexplained pulmonary hypertension in chronic myeloproliferative disorders. *Chest* 2001; 120:801.

[129] Cortelezzi A, Gritti G, Del Papa N, et al. Pulmonary arterial hypertension in primary myelofibrosis is common and associated with an altered angiogenic status. *Leukemia* 2008; 22:646.

[130] Vaa BE, Wolanskyj AP, Roeker L, et al. Pruritus in primary myelofibrosis: clinical and laboratory correlates. *Am J Hematol* 2012; 87:136.

[131] O'Reilly RA. Splenomegaly in 2,505 patients in a large university medical center from 1913 to 1995. 1913 to 1962: 2,056 patients. *West J Med* 1998; 169:78.

[132] Lichtman MA. Idiopathic myelofibrosis (agnogenic myeloid metaplasia). In: *Williams' Hematology,* 5th ed, Beutler E, Lichtman MA, Coller BS, Kipps TJ (Eds), McGraw-Hill, New York 1995. p.331.

[133] Georgiades CS, Neyman EG, Francis IR, et al. Typical and atypical presentations of extramedullary hemopoiesis. *AJR Am J Roentgenol* 2002; 179:1239.

[134] Koch CA, Li CY, Mesa RA, Tefferi A. Nonhepatosplenic extramedullary hematopoiesis: associated diseases, pathology, clinical course, and treatment. *Mayo Clin Proc* 2003; 78:1223.

[135] Bartlett RP, Greipp PR, Tefferi A, et al. Extramedullary hematopoiesis manifesting as a symptomatic pleural effusion. *Mayo Clin Proc* 1995; 70:1161.

[136] Knobel B, Melamud E, Virag I, Meytes D. Ectopic medullary hematopoiesis as a cause of ascites in agnogenic myeloid metaplasia. Case report and review of the literature. *Acta Haematol* 1993; 89:104.

[137] Lioté F, Yeni P, Teillet-Thiebaud F, et al. Ascites revealing peritoneal and hepatic extramedullary hematopoiesis with peliosis in agnogenic myeloid metaplasia: case report and review of the literature. *Am J Med* 1991; 90:111.

[138] Yusen RD, Kollef MH. Acute respiratory failure due to extramedullary hematopoiesis. *Chest* 1995; 108:1170.

[139] Richters ML. Myelofibrosis, diffuse alveolar hemorrhage and radiation treatment. *Am J Hematol* 2013; 88:922.

[140] Lundh B, Brandt L, Cronqvist S, Eyrich R. Intracranial myeloid metaplasia in myelofibrosis. *Scand J Haematol* 1982; 28:91.

[141] Koch BL, Bisset GS 3rd, Bisset RR, Zimmer MB. Intracranial extramedullary hematopoiesis: MR findings with pathologic correlation. *AJR Am J Roentgenol* 1994; 162:1419.

[142] Loewy G, Mathew A, Distenfeld A. Skin manifestation of agnogenic myeloid metaplasia. *Am J Hematol* 1994; 45:167.

[143] Pecci A, Croci G, Balduini CL, Boveri E. Cutaneous involvement by post-polycythemia vera myelofibrosis. *Am J Hematol* 2013.

[144] Fedeli G, Certo M, Cannizzaro O, et al. Extramedullary hematopoiesis involving the esophagus in myelofibrosis. *Am J Gastroenterol* 1990; 85:1512.

[145] Schreibman D, Brenner B, Jacobs R, et al. Small intestinal myeloid metaplasia. *JAMA* 1988; 259:2580.

[146] Thiele J, Kvasnicka HM, Werden C, et al. Idiopathic primary osteo-myelofibrosis: a clinico-pathological study on 208 patients with special emphasis on evolution of disease features, differentiation from essential thrombocythemia and variables of prognostic impact. *Leuk Lymphoma* 1996; 22:303.

[147] Beer PA, Campbell PJ, Green AR. Comparison of different criteria for the diagnosis of primary myelofibrosis reveals limited clinical utility for measurement of serum lactate dehydrogenase. *Haematologica* 2010; 95:1960.

[148] Thiele J, Kvasnicka HM, Facchetti F, et al. European consensus on grading bone marrow fibrosis and assessment of cellularity. *Haematologica* 2005; 90:1128.

[149] Tefferi A, Thiele J, Orazi A, et al. Proposals and rationale for revision of the World Health Organization diagnostic criteria for polycythemia vera, essential thrombocythemia, and primary myelofibrosis: recommendations from an ad hoc international expert panel. *Blood* 2007; 110:1092.

[150] Vener C, Fracchiolla NS, Gianelli U, et al. Prognostic implications of the European consensus for grading of bone marrow fibrosis in chronic idiopathic myelofibrosis. *Blood* 2008; 111:1862.

[151] Landaw SA. Tissue imaging and cell survival studies for evaluating patients with hematologic disorders. In: *Williams' Hematology,* 5th ed, Beutler E, Lichtman MA, Coller B, et al. (Eds), McGraw-Hill, New York 1995. p.L12.

[152] Tefferi A, Lasho TL, Schwager SM, et al. The JAK2(V617F) tyrosine kinase mutation in myelofibrosis with myeloid metaplasia: lineage specificity and clinical correlates. *Br J Haematol* 2005; 131:320.

[153] Mesa RA, Li CY, Ketterling RP, et al. Leukemic transformation in myelofibrosis with myeloid metaplasia: a single-institution experience with 91 cases. *Blood* 2005; 105:973.

[154] Cervantes F, Tassies D, Salgado C, et al. Acute transformation in nonleukemic chronic myeloproliferative disorders: actuarial probability and main characteristics in a series of 218 patients. *Acta Haematol* 1991; 85:124.

[155] Ragni MV, Shreiner DP. Spontaneous "remission' of agnogenic myeloid metaplasia and termination in acute myeloid leukemia. *Arch Intern Med* 1981; 141:1481.

[156] Hernández JM, San Miguel JF, González M, et al. Development of acute leukaemia after idiopathic myelofibrosis. *J Clin Pathol* 1992; 45:427.

[157] Passamonti F, Rumi E, Elena C, et al. Incidence of leukaemia in patients with primary myelofibrosis and RBC-transfusion-dependence. *Br J Haematol* 2010; 150:719.

[158] Huang J, Li CY, Mesa RA, et al. Risk factors for leukemic transformation in patients with primary myelofibrosis. *Cancer* 2008; 112:2726.

[159] Tefferi A, Thiele J, Orazi A, et al. Proposals and rationale for revision of the World Health Organization diagnostic criteria for polycythemia vera, essential thrombocythemia, and primary myelofibrosis: recommendations from an ad hoc international expert panel. *Blood* 2007; 110:1092.

[160] Tefferi A, Skoda R, Vardiman JW. Myeloproliferative neoplasms: contemporary diagnosis using histology and genetics. *Nat Rev Clin Oncol* 2009; 6:627.

[161] Barosi G, Mesa RA, Thiele J, et al. Proposed criteria for the diagnosis of post-polycythemia vera and post-essential thrombocythemia myelofibrosis: a consensus statement from the International Working Group for Myelofibrosis Research and Treatment. *Leukemia* 2008; 22:437.

[162] Thiele J, Kvasnicka HM, Werden C, et al. Idiopathic primary osteo-myelofibrosis: a clinico-pathological study on 208 patients with special emphasis on evolution of disease features, differentiation from essential thrombocythemia and variables of prognostic impact. *Leuk Lymphoma* 1996; 22:303.

[163] Dekmezian R, Kantarjian HM, Keating MJ, et al. The relevance of reticulin stain-measured fibrosis at diagnosis in chronic myelogenous leukemia. *Cancer* 1987; 59:1739.

[164] Singh M, Bofinger A, Taylor K, Ba Pe R. Myelodysplasia with myelofibrosis--a distinct subgroup within the myelodysplastic syndromes. *Pathology* 1994; 26:69.

[165] Vallespí T, Imbert M, Mecucci C, et al. Diagnosis, classification, and cytogenetics of myelodysplastic syndromes. *Haematologica* 1998; 83:258.

[166] Poulsen LW, Melsen F, Bendix K. A histomorphometric study of haematological disorders with respect to marrow fibrosis and osteosclerosis. *APMIS* 1998; 106:495.

[167] Georgii A, Buhr T, Buesche G, et al. Classification and staging of Ph-negative myeloproliferative disorders by histopathology from bone marrow biopsies. *Leuk Lymphoma* 1996; 22 Suppl 1:15.

[168] Dameshek W. Some speculations on the myeloproliferative disorders. *Blood* 1951; 6:372.

[169] Thiele J, Kvasnicka HM, Müllauer L, et al. Essential thrombocythemia versus early primary myelofibrosis: a multicenter study to validate the WHO classification. *Blood* 2011; 117:5710.

[170] Cervantes F, Dupriez B, Pereira A, et al. New prognostic scoring system for primary myelofibrosis based on a study of the International Working Group for Myelofibrosis Research and Treatment. *Blood* 2009; 113:2895.

[171] Hussein K, Huang J, Lasho T, et al. Karyotype complements the International Prognostic Scoring System for primary myelofibrosis. *Eur J Haematol* 2009; 82:255.

[172] Tefferi A, Meyer RG, Wyatt WA, Dewald GW. Comparison of peripheral blood interphase cytogenetics with bone marrow karyotype analysis in myelofibrosis with myeloid metaplasia. *Br J Haematol* 2001; 115:316.

[173] Tam CS, Abruzzo LV, Lin KI, et al. The role of cytogenetic abnormalities as a prognostic marker in primary myelofibrosis: applicability at the time of diagnosis and later during disease course. *Blood* 2009; 113:4171.

[174] Hussein K, Pardanani AD, Van Dyke DL, et al. International Prognostic Scoring System-independent cytogenetic risk categorization in primary myelofibrosis. *Blood* 2010; 115:496.

[175] Caramazza D, Begna KH, Gangat N, et al. Refined cytogenetic-risk categorization for overall and leukemia-free survival in primary myelofibrosis: a single center study of 433 patients. *Leukemia* 2011; 25:82.

[176] Tefferi A, Siragusa S, Hussein K, et al. Transfusion-dependency at presentation and its acquisition in the first year of diagnosis are both equally detrimental for survival in primary myelofibrosis--prognostic relevance is independent of IPSS or karyotype. *Am J Hematol* 2010; 85:14.

[177] Patnaik MM, Caramazza D, Gangat N, et al. Age and platelet count are IPSS-independent prognostic factors in young patients with primary myelofibrosis and complement IPSS in predicting very long or very short survival. *Eur J Haematol* 2010; 84:105.

[178] Gangat N, Caramazza D, Vaidya R, et al. DIPSS plus: a refined Dynamic International Prognostic Scoring System for primary myelofibrosis that incorporates prognostic information from karyotype, platelet count, and transfusion status. *J Clin Oncol* 2011; 29:392.

[179] Tefferi A, Lasho TL, Jimma T, et al. One thousand patients with primary myelofibrosis: the mayo clinic experience. *Mayo Clin Proc* 2012; 87:25.

[180] Cervantes F, Barosi G, Demory JL, et al. Myelofibrosis with myeloid metaplasia in young individuals: disease characteristics, prognostic factors and identification of risk groups. *Br J Haematol* 1998; 102:684.

[181] Guardiola P, Anderson JE, Bandini G, et al. Allogeneic stem cell transplantation for agnogenic myeloid metaplasia: a European Group for Blood and Marrow Transplantation, Société Française de Greffe de Moelle, Gruppo Italiano per il Trapianto del Midollo Osseo, and Fred Hutchinson Cancer Research Center Collaborative Study. *Blood* 1999; 93:2831.

[182] Barbui T, Barosi G, Birgegard G, et al. Philadelphia-negative classical myeloproliferative neoplasms: critical concepts and management recommendations from European LeukemiaNet. *J Clin Oncol* 2011; 29:761.

[183] Arana-Yi C, Quintás-Cardama A, Giles F, et al. Advances in the therapy of chronic idiopathic myelofibrosis. *Oncologist* 2006; 11:929.

[184] Maziarz RT, Mesa RA, Tefferi A. Allogeneic stem cell transplantation for chronic myeloproliferative disorders and myelodysplastic syndromes: the question is "when?". *Mayo Clin Proc* 2003; 78:941.

[185] Babushok D, Hexner E. Allogeneic transplantation for myelofibrosis: for whom, when, and what are the true benefits? *Curr Opin Hematol* 2014; 21:114.

[186] Robin M, Tabrizi R, Mohty M, et al. Allogeneic haematopoietic stem cell transplantation for myelofibrosis: a report of the Société Française de Greffe de Moelle et de Thérapie Cellulaire (SFGM-TC). *Br J Haematol* 2011; 152:331.

[187] Guardiola P, Anderson JE, Bandini G, et al. Allogeneic stem cell transplantation for agnogenic myeloid metaplasia: a European Group for Blood and Marrow Transplantation, Société Française de Greffe de Moelle, Gruppo Italiano per il Trapianto del Midollo Osseo, and Fred Hutchinson Cancer Research Center Collaborative Study. *Blood* 1999; 93:2831.

[188] Guardiola P, Anderson JE, Gluckman E. Myelofibrosis with myeloid metaplasia. *N Engl J Med* 2000; 343:659; author reply 659.

[189] Samuelson S, Sandmaier BM, Heslop HE, et al. Allogeneic haematopoietic cell transplantation for myelofibrosis in 30 patients 60-78 years of age. *Br J Haematol* 2011; 153.

[190] Kröger N, Holler E, Kobbe G, et al. Allogeneic stem cell transplantation after reduced-intensity conditioning in patients with myelofibrosis: a prospective, multicenter study of the Chronic Leukemia Working Party of the European Group for Blood and Marrow Transplantation. *Blood* 2009; 114:5264.

[191] Alchalby H, Badbaran A, Zabelina T, et al. Impact of JAK2V617F mutation status, allele burden, and clearance after allogeneic stem cell transplantation for myelofibrosis. *Blood* 2010; 116:3572.

[192] Devine SM, Hoffman R, Verma A, et al. Allogeneic blood cell transplantation following reduced-intensity conditioning is effective therapy for older patients with myelofibrosis with myeloid metaplasia. *Blood* 2002; 99:2255.

[193] Hessling J, Kröger N, Werner M, et al. Dose-reduced conditioning regimen followed by allogeneic stem cell transplantation in patients with myelofibrosis with myeloid metaplasia. *Br J Haematol* 2002; 119:769.

[194] Kröger N, Zabelina T, Schieder H, et al. Pilot study of reduced-intensity conditioning followed by allogeneic stem cell transplantation from related and unrelated donors in patients with myelofibrosis. *Br J Haematol* 2005; 128:690.

[195] Rondelli D, Barosi G, Bacigalupo A, et al. Allogeneic hematopoietic stem-cell transplantation with reduced-intensity conditioning in intermediate- or high-risk patients with myelofibrosis with myeloid metaplasia. *Blood* 2005; 105:4115.

[196] Kröger N, Holler E, Kobbe G, et al. Allogeneic stem cell transplantation after reduced-intensity conditioning in patients with myelofibrosis: a prospective, multicenter study of the Chronic Leukemia Working Party of the European Group for Blood and Marrow Transplantation. *Blood* 2009; 114:5264.

[197] Bacigalupo A, Soraru M, Dominietto A, et al. Allogeneic hemopoietic SCT for patients with primary myelofibrosis: a predictive transplant score based on transfusion requirement, spleen size and donor type. *Bone Marrow Transplant* 2010; 45:458.

[198] Abelsson J, Merup M, Birgegård G, et al. The outcome of allo-HSCT for 92 patients with myelofibrosis in the Nordic countries. *Bone Marrow Transplant* 2012; 47:380.

[199] Alchalby H, Yunus DR, Zabelina T, et al. Risk models predicting survival after reduced-intensity transplantation for myelofibrosis. *Br J Haematol* 2012; 157:75.

[200] siren" "S," lash "TL," Hanson "CA," et "al." The presence of JAK2V617F in primary myelofibrosis or its allele burden in polycythemia very predicts "chem sensitivity" to "hydroxyurea." *Am J hepatol* "2008;" "83:363".

[201] Harrison C, Kiladjian JJ, Al-Ali HK, et al. JAK inhibition with ruxolitinib versus best available therapy for myelofibrosis. *N Engl J Med* 2012; 366:787.

[202] Verstovsek S, Mesa RA, Gotlib J, et al. A double-blind, placebo-controlled trial of ruxolitinib for myelofibrosis. *N Engl J Med* 2012; 366:799.

[203] Tefferi A, Pardanani A. Serious adverse events during ruxolitinib treatment discontinuation in patients with myelofibrosis. *Mayo Clin Proc* 2011; 86:1188

[204] Dai T, Friedman EW, Barta SK. Ruxolitinib withdrawal syndrome leading to tumor lysis. *J Clin Oncol* 2013; 31:e430.

[205] The JAK-inhibitor ruxolitinib impairs dendritic cell function in vitro and in vivo. *Blood* 2013; 122:1192.

[206] Gilbert HS. Long term treatment of myeloproliferative disease with interferon-alpha-2b: feasibility and efficacy. *Cancer* 1998; 83:1205.

[207] Mesa RA, Elliott MA, Schroeder G, Tefferi A. Durable responses to thalidomide-based drug therapy for myelofibrosis with myeloid metaplasia. *Mayo Clin Proc* 2004; 79:883.

[208] Mesa RA, Steensma DP, Pardanani A, et al. A phase 2 trial of combination low-dose thalidomide and prednisone for the treatment of myelofibrosis with myeloid metaplasia. *Blood* 2003; 101:2534.

[209] Merup M, Kutti J, Birgergård G, et al. Negligible clinical effects of thalidomide in patients with myelofibrosis with myeloid metaplasia. *Med Oncol* 2002; 19:79.

[210] Tefferi A, Cortes J, Verstovsek S, et al. Lenalidomide therapy in myelofibrosis with myeloid metaplasia. *Blood* 2006; 108:1158.

[211] Tefferi A, Verstovsek S, Barosi G, et al. Pomalidomide is active in the treatment of anemia associated with myelofibrosis. *J Clin Oncol* 2009; 27:4563.

[212] Steensma DP, Mesa RA, Li CY, et al. Etanercept, a soluble tumor necrosis factor receptor, palliates constitutional symptoms in patients with myelofibrosis with myeloid metaplasia: results of a pilot study. *Blood* 2002; 99:2252.

[213] Guglielmelli P, Barosi G, Rambaldi A, et al. Safety and efficacy of everolimus, a mTOR inhibitor, as single agent in a phase 1/2 study in patients with myelofibrosis. *Blood* 2011; 118:2069.

[214] Quintás-Cardama A, Kantarjian H, Estrov Z, et al. Therapy with the histone deacetylase inhibitor pracinostat for patients with myelofibrosis. *Leuk Res* 2012; 36:1124.

[215] Rambaldi A, Dellacasa CM, Finazzi G, et al. A pilot study of the Histone-Deacetylase inhibitor Givinostat in patients with JAK2V617F positive chronic myeloproliferative neoplasms. *Br J Haematol* 2010; 150:446.

[216] Mascarenhas J, Lu M, Li T, et al. A phase I study of panobinostat (LBH589) in patients with primary myelofibrosis (PMF) and post-polycythaemia vera/essential thrombocythaemia myelofibrosis (post-PV/ET MF). *Br J Haematol* 2013; 161:68.

[217] DeAngelo DJ, Mesa RA, Fiskus W, et al. Phase II trial of panobinostat, an oral pan-deacetylase inhibitor in patients with primary myelofibrosis, post-essential thrombocythaemia, and post-polycythaemia vera myelofibrosis. *Br J Haematol* 2013; 162:326.

[218] Benbassat J, Penchas S, Ligumski M. Splenectomy in patients with agnogenic myeloid metaplasia: an analysis of 321 published cases. *Br J Haematol* 1979; 42:207.

[219] Mesa RA, Nagorney DS, Schwager S, et al. Palliative goals, patient selection, and perioperative platelet management: outcomes and lessons from 3 decades of splenectomy for myelofibrosis with myeloid metaplasia at the Mayo Clinic. *Cancer* 2006; 107:361.

[220] Barosi G, Ambrosetti A, Buratti A, et al. Splenectomy for patients with myelofibrosis with myeloid metaplasia: pretreatment variables and outcome prediction. Leukemia 1993; 7:200.

[221] Faoro LN, Tefferi A, Mesa RA. Long-term analysis of the palliative benefit of 2-chlorodeoxyadenosine for myelofibrosis with myeloid metaplasia. *Eur J Haematol* 2005; 74:117.

[222] Barosi G, Ambrosetti A, Centra A, et al. Splenectomy and risk of blast transformation in myelofibrosis with myeloid metaplasia. Italian Cooperative Study Group on Myeloid with Myeloid Metaplasia. *Blood* 1998; 91:3630.

[223] Elliott MA, Chen MG, Silverstein MN, Tefferi A. Splenic irradiation for symptomatic splenomegaly associated with myelofibrosis with myeloid metaplasia. *Br J Haematol* 1998; 103:505

[224] Harrison CN. Current trends in essential thrombocythaemia. *Br J Haematol* 2002; 117:796.

[225] Schafer AI. Thrombocytosis. *N Engl J Med* 2004; 350:1211.

[226] Ma X, Vanasse G, Cartmel B, et al. Prevalence of polycythemia vera and essential thrombocythemia. *Am J Hematol* 2008; 83:359.

[227] Mesa RA, Silverstein MN, Jacobsen SJ, et al. Population-based incidence and survival figures in essential thrombocythemia and agnogenic myeloid metaplasia: an Olmsted County Study, 1976-1995. *Am J Hematol* 1999; 61:10.

[228] Bellucci S, Janvier M, Tobelem G, et al. Essential thrombocythemias. Clinical evolutionary and biological data. *Cancer* 1986; 58:2440.

[229] Gugliotta L, et al. Epidemiological, diagnostic, therapeutic, and prognostic aspects of essential thrombocythemia in a retrospective study of the GIMMC group in two thousand patients. *Blood* 1997; 90:348a.

[230] Hasle H, Wadsworth LD, Massing BG, et al. A population-based study of childhood myelodysplastic syndrome in British Columbia, Canada. *Br J Haematol* 1999; 106:1027.

[231] Hasle H, Kerndrup G, Jacobsen BB. Childhood myelodysplastic syndrome in Denmark: incidence and predisposing conditions. *Leukemia* 1995; 9:1569.

[232] Giona F, Teofili L, Moleti ML, et al. Thrombocythemia and polycythemia in patients younger than 20 years at diagnosis: clinical and biologic features, treatment, and long-term outcome. *Blood* 2012; 119:2219.

[233] Pardanani AD, Levine RL, Lasho T, et al. MPL515 mutations in myeloproliferative and other myeloid disorders: a study of 1182 patients. *Blood* 2006; 108:3472.

[234] Kiladjian JJ, Elkassar N, Hetet G, et al. Study of the thrombopoitin receptor in essential thrombocythemia. *Leukemia* 1997; 11:1821.

[235] Taksin AL, Couedic JP, Dusanter-Fourt I, et al. Autonomous megakaryocyte growth in essential thrombocythemia and idiopathic myelofibrosis is not related to a c-mpl mutation or to an autocrine stimulation by Mpl-L. *Blood* 1999; 93:125.

[236] El-Kassar N, Hetet G, Brière J, Grandchamp B. Clonality analysis of hematopoiesis and thrombopoietin levels in patients with essential thrombocythemia. *Leuk Lymphoma* 1998; 30:181.

[237] Griesshammer M, Hornkohl A, Nichol JL, et al. High levels of thrombopoietin in sera of patients with essential thrombocythemia:

cause or consequence of abnormal platelet production? *Ann Hematol* 1998; 77:211.

[238] Hirayama Y, Sakamaki S, Matsunaga T, et al. Concentrations of thrombopoietin in bone marrow in normal subjects and in patients with idiopathic thrombocytopenic purpura, aplastic anemia, and essential thrombocythemia correlate with its mRNA expression of bone marrow stromal cells. *Blood* 1998; 92:46.

[239] Horikawa Y, Matsumura I, Hashimoto K, et al. Markedly reduced expression of platelet c-mpl receptor in essential thrombocythemia. *Blood* 1997; 90:4031.

[240] Fialkow PJ, Faguet GB, Jacobson RJ, et al. Evidence that essential thrombocythemia is a clonal disorder with origin in a multipotent stem cell. *Blood* 1981; 58:916.

[241] El-Kassar N, Hetet G, Brière J, Grandchamp B. Clonality analysis of hematopoiesis and thrombopoietin levels in patients with essential thrombocythemia. *Leuk Lymphoma* 1998; 30:181.

[242] el-Kassar N, Hetet G, Brière J, Grandchamp B. Clonality analysis of hematopoiesis in essential thrombocythemia: advantages of studying T lymphocytes and platelets. *Blood* 1997; 89:128.

[243] Janssen JW, Anger BR, Drexler HG, et al. Essential thrombocythemia in two sisters originating from different stem cell levels. *Blood* 1990; 75:1633

[244] Chen GL, Prchal JT. X-linked clonality testing: interpretation and limitations. *Blood* 2007; 110:1411.

[245] Chen GL, Prchal JT. X-linked clonality testing: interpretation and limitations. *Blood* 2007; 110:1411.

[246] Champion KM, Gilbert JG, Asimakopoulos FA, et al. Clonal haemopoiesis in normal elderly women: implications for the myeloproliferative disorders and myelodysplastic syndromes. *Br J Haematol* 1997; 97:920

[247] Harrison CN, Gale RE, Machin SJ, Linch DC. A large proportion of patients with a diagnosis of essential thrombocythemia do not have a clonal disorder and may be at lower risk of thrombotic complications. *Blood* 1999; 93:417.

[248] Schafer AI. Molecular basis of the diagnosis and treatment of polycythemia vera and essential thrombocythemia. Blood 2006; 107:4214.

[249] Fenaux P, Simon M, Caulier MT, et al. Clinical course of essential thrombocythemia in 147 cases. *Cancer* 1990; 66:549.

[250] Chistolini A, Mazzucconi MG, Ferrari A, et al. Essential thrombocythemia: a retrospective study on the clinical course of 100 patients. *Haematologica* 1990; 75:537.

[251] Cortelazzo S, Viero P, Finazzi G, et al. Incidence and risk factors for thrombotic complications in a historical cohort of 100 patients with essential thrombocythemia. *J Clin Oncol* 1990; 8:556.

[252] Fenaux P, Simon M, Caulier MT, et al. Clinical course of essential thrombocythemia in 147 cases. *Cancer* 1990; 66:549.

[253] Bellucci S, Janvier M, Tobelem G, et al. Essential thrombocythemias. Clinical evolutionary and biological data. *Cancer* 1986; 58:2440.

[254] Gugliotta L, et al. Epidemiological, diagnostic, therapeutic, and prognostic aspects of essential thrombocythemia in a retrospective study of the GIMMC group in two thousand patients. *Blood* 1997; 90:348a.

[255] Chistolini A, Mazzucconi MG, Ferrari A, et al. Essential thrombocythemia: a retrospective study on the clinical course of 100 patients. *Haematologica* 1990; 75:537.

[256] Colombi M, Radaelli F, Zocchi L, Maiolo AT. Thrombotic and hemorrhagic complications in essential thrombocythemia. A retrospective study of 103 patients. *Cancer* 1991; 67:2926.

[257] Carobbio A, Thiele J, Passamonti F, et al. Risk factors for arterial and venous thrombosis in WHO-defined essential thrombocythemia: an international study of 891 patients. *Blood* 2011; 117:5857.

[258] Gangat N, Wolanskyj AP, Schwager SM, et al. Estrogen-based hormone therapy and thrombosis risk in women with essential thrombocythemia. *Cancer* 2006; 106:2406.

[259] Carobbio A, Thiele J, Passamonti F, et al. Risk factors for arterial and venous thrombosis in WHO-defined essential thrombocythemia: an international study of 891 patients. *Blood* 2011; 117:5857.

[260] Colombi M, Radaelli F, Zocchi L, Maiolo AT. Thrombotic and hemorrhagic complications in essential thrombocythemia. A retrospective study of 103 patients. *Cancer* 1991; 67:2926.

[261] Cervantes F, Tassies D, Salgado C, et al. Acute transformation in nonleukemic chronic myeloproliferative disorders: actuarial probability and main characteristics in a series of 218 patients. *Acta Haematol* 1991; 85:124.

[262] Griesshammer M, Heimpel H, Pearson TC. Essential thrombocythemia and pregnancy. *Leuk Lymphoma* 1996; 22 Suppl 1:57.

[263] Passamonti F, Randi ML, Rumi E, et al. Increased risk of pregnancy complications in patients with essential thrombocythemia carrying the JAK2 (617V>F) mutation. *Blood* 2007; 110:485.

[264] Pagliaro P, Arrigoni L, Muggiasca ML, et al. Primary thrombocythemia and pregnancy: treatment and outcome in fifteen cases. *Am J Hematol* 1996; 53:6.

[265] Picardi M, Martinelli V, Ciancia R, et al. Measurement of spleen volume by ultrasound scanning in patients with thrombocytosis: a prospective study. *Blood* 2002; 99:4228.

[266] Murphy S, Peterson P, Iland H, Laszlo J. Experience of the Polycythemia Vera Study Group with essential thrombocythemia: a final report on diagnostic criteria, survival, and leukemic transition by treatment. *Semin Hematol 1997*; 34:29.

[267] Campbell PJ, Scott LM, Buck G, et al. Definition of subtypes of essential thrombocythaemia and relation to polycythaemia vera based on JAK2 V617F mutation status: a prospective study. *Lancet* 2005; 366:1945.

[268] Gangat N, Wolanskyj AP, McClure RF, et al. Risk stratification for survival and leukemic transformation in essential thrombocythemia: a single institutional study of 605 patients. *Leukemia* 2007; 21:270.

[269] Rumi E, Pietra D, Ferretti V, et al. JAK2 or CALR mutation status defines subtypes of essential thrombocythemia with substantially different clinical course and outcomes. *Blood* 2013.

[270] Rotunno G, Mannarelli C, Guglielmelli P, et al. Impact of calreticulin mutations on clinical and hematological phenotype and outcome in essential thrombocythemia. *Blood* 2013.

[271] Nangalia J, Massie CE, Baxter EJ, et al. Somatic CALR mutations in myeloproliferative neoplasms with nonmutated JAK2. *N Engl J Med* 2013; 369:2391.

[272] Klampfl T, Gisslinger H, Harutyunyan AS, et al. Somatic mutations of calreticulin in myeloproliferative neoplasms. *N Engl J Med* 2013; 369:2379.

[273] Wolanskyj AP, Lasho TL, Schwager SM, et al. JAK2 mutation in essential thrombocythaemia: clinical associations and long-term prognostic relevance. *Br J Haematol* 2005; 131:208.

[274] Cheung B, Radia D, Pantelidis P, ct al. The presence of the JAK2 V617F mutation is associated with a higher haemoglobin and increased risk of thrombosis in essential thrombocythaemia. *Br J Haematol* 2006; 132:244.

[275] Kittur J, Knudson RA, Lasho TL, et al. Clinical correlates of JAK2V617F allele burden in essential thrombocythemia. *Cancer* 2007; 109:2279.

[276] Zhang S, Qiu H, Fischer BS, et al. JAK2 V617F patients with essential thrombocythemia present with clinical features of polycythemia vera. *Leuk Lymphoma* 2008; 49:696.

[277] Toyama K, Karasawa M, Yamane A, et al. JAK2-V617F mutation analysis of granulocytes and platelets from patients with chronic myeloproliferative disorders: advantage of studying platelets. *Br J Haematol* 2007; 139:64.

[278] Wong RS, Cheng CK, Chan NP, et al. JAK2 V617F mutation is associated with increased risk of thrombosis in Chinese patients with essential thrombocythaemia. *Br J Haematol* 2008; 141:902.

[279] Chao MP, Gotlib J. Two faces of ET: CALR and JAK2. *Blood* 2014; 123:1438.

[280] Passamonti F, Thiele J, Girodon F, et al. A prognostic model to predict survival in 867 World Health Organization-defined essential thrombocythemia at diagnosis: a study by the International Working Group on Myelofibrosis Research and Treatment. *Blood* 2012; 120:1197.

[281] Gangat N, Wolanskyj AP, McClure RF, et al. Risk stratification for survival and leukemic transformation in essential thrombocythemia: a single institutional study of 605 patients. *Leukemia* 2007; 21:270.

[282] Barbui T, Finazzi G, Carobbio A, et al. Development and validation of an International Prognostic Score of thrombosis in World Health Organization-essential thrombocythemia (IPSET-thrombosis). *Blood* 2012; 120:5128.

[283] Cortelazzo S, Viero P, Finazzi G, et al. Incidence and risk factors for thrombotic complications in a historical cohort of 100 patients with essential thrombocythemia. *J Clin Oncol* 1990; 8:556.

[284] van Genderen PJ, Mulder PG, Waleboer M, et al. Prevention and treatment of thrombotic complications in essential thrombocythaemia: efficacy and safety of aspirin. *Br J Haematol* 1997; 97:179.

[285] Patrono C, Rocca B, De Stefano V. Platelet activation and inhibition in polycythemia vera and essential thrombocythemia. *Blood* 2013; 121:1701.

[286] Michiels JJ, Koudstaal PJ, Mulder AH, van Vliet HH. Transient neurologic and ocular manifestations in primary thrombocythemia. *Neurology* 1993; 43:1107.

[287] Michiels JJ, Abels J, Steketee J, et al. Erythromelalgia caused by platelet-mediated arteriolar inflammation and thrombosis in thrombocythemia. *Ann Intern Med* 1985; 102:466.

[288] Antonioli E, Guglielmelli P, Pieri L, et al. Hydroxyurea-related toxicity in 3,411 patients with Ph'-negative MPN. *Am J Hematol* 2012; 87:552.

[289] Hernández-Boluda JC, Alvarez-Larrán A, Gómez M, et al. Clinical evaluation of the European LeukaemiaNet criteria for clinicohaematological response and resistance/intolerance to hydroxycarbamide in essential thrombocythaemia. *Br J Haematol* 2011; 152:81.

[290] Mazur EM, Rosmarin AG, Sohl PA, et al. Analysis of the mechanism of anagrelide-induced thrombocytopenia in humans. *Blood* 1992; 79:1931.

[291] Tomer A. Effects of anagrelide on in vivo megakaryocyte proliferation and maturation in essential thrombocythemia. *Blood* 2002; 99:1602.

[292] Balduini CL, Bertolino G, Noris P, Ascari E. Effect of anagrelide on platelet count and function in patients with thrombocytosis and myeloproliferative disorders. *Haematologica* 1992; 77:40.

[293] Storen EC, Tefferi A. Long-term use of anagrelide in young patients with essential thrombocythemia. *Blood* 2001; 97:863.

[294] Jurgens DJ, Moreno-Aspitia A, Tefferi A. Anagrelide-associated cardiomyopathy in polycythemia vera and essential thrombocythemia. *Haematologica* 2004; 89:1394.

[295] Amabile CM, Spencer AP. Keeping your patient with heart failure safe: a review of potentially dangerous medications. *Arch Intern Med* 2004; 164:709.

[296] Campbell PJ, Bareford D, Erber WN, et al. Reticulin accumulation in essential thrombocythemia: prognostic significance and relationship to therapy. *J Clin Oncol* 2009; 27:2991.

[297] Sacchi S, Gugliotta L, Papineschi F, et al. Alfa-interferon in the treatment of essential thrombocythemia: clinical results and evaluation of its biological effects on the hematopoietic neoplastic clone. Italian Cooperative Group on ET. *Leukemia* 1998; 12:289.

[298] Greist A. The role of blood component removal in essential and reactive thrombocytosis. *Ther Apher* 2002; 6:36.

[299] Tefferi A. Risk-based management in essential thrombocythemia. ASH Education Program Book. *Hematology* 1999:172.

In: Myeloproliferative Disorders
Editor: Anthony M. Camden

ISBN: 978-1-63321-201-5
© 2014 Nova Science Publishers, Inc.

Chapter 2

HISTOPATHOLOGY AND DIAGNOSTIC APPROACHES TO THE MYELOPROLIFERATIVE NEOPLASMS

Christina Salazar[1], Sanjeev M. Balamohan[1], Patrick D. Millikan[1], Wendy H. Raskind[2] and Melissa A. Kacena[1]

[1]Department of Orthopaedic Surgery,
Indiana University School of Medicine
[2]University of Washington School of Medicine, WA, US

ABSTRACT

Myeloproliferative neoplasms (MPNs) are diseases in which clonal cells of one or more myeloid lineages proliferate in the bone marrow. Elevated megakaryopoeisis is prominent among these disorders and contributes to essential thrombocythemia, primary myelofibrosis, polycythemia vera, and chronic myelogenous leukemia, which are considered the most common MPNs. Acute megakaryoblastic leukemia is also characterized by expansion of the megarkaryocytic lineage. The diseases all share a similar clinical course, often exhibiting splenomegaly, hepatomegaly, thrombocytosis, and various clotting and bleeding symptoms. The similarity of symptoms necessitates a combination of histological, clinical, and cytogenetic tests in order to make an accurate diagnosis. The V617 JAK2 mutation has been identified in most patients with polycythemia vera, and is also present in a subset of patients with essential thrombocythemia and primary myelofibrosis. Novel mutations are also being studied for their relevance to the pathogenesis of MPNs and may allow for further differentiation of the diseases. However, bone marrow histopathology may still serve as the most discriminating method to diagnose these disorders. The MPNs all display distinct megakaryocyte morphology and the bone marrow histopathology allows for investigation of proliferation of other hematopoietic lineages.

INTRODUCTION

The concept of myeloproliferative disorders was originally proposed by William Dameshek in 1951 [1] when he described essential thrombocythemia, primary myelofibrosis, polycythemia vera, chronic myelogenous leukemia, and erythroleukemia. The former four, all chronic diseases, came to be considered "classic" myeloproliferative diseases while the latter one was subsequently reclassified as an acute myeloid leukemia [2]. The broader classification of chronic myeloproliferative diseases, as defined by the World Health Organization (WHO) in 2008, includes these four diseases as well as chronic neutrophilic leukemia, chronic eosinophilic leukemia, mast cell disease, and "unclassifiable" myeloproliferative disease. The WHO also gave chronic myeloproliferative diseases the new term myeloproliferative neoplasms (MPNs) [3]. This chapter focuses on the MPNs that are mostly or partially characterized by proliferation of the megakaryocyte (MK) lineage, which happen to be the four classic myeloproliferative disorders. Not only do all four exhibit prominent megakaryopoiesis, but the MKs in each disease display distinct morphologies that are evident by histological analysis. Our group studies MKs as well as phenotypes resulting from GATA-1 mutations, and among these are transient myeloproliferative disorder and acute megakaryoblastic leukemia [4]. These diseases tend to manifest in infants with trisomy 21. While not technically considered MPNs, they nonetheless exhibit proliferation of MK lineage cells which display a unique morphology. Thus, this chapter also reviews these two disorders. Distinctions between the six reviewed diseases will be drawn based on histopathology (with an emphasis on the MK lineage), various other diagnostic criteria, clinical manifestations, and cytogenetics.

ESSENTIAL THROMBOCYTHEMIA

Histolopathology

MKs as well as their nuclei are enlarged in Essential Thrombocythemia (ET) [5-9]. One of the distinctive features is that the nuclei (sometimes described as staghorn-like) possess high numbers of deep lobules. MKs in ET are distinguished from those in other MPNs primarily by the increased segmentation of their nuclei [10]. MK morphology is fairly consistent, characteristically lacking pleomorphy. The cytoplasm is mature and the cells lack any disturbance of the nuclear-cytoplasmic ratio [11]. High levels of MK proliferation are seen in ET. Unlike other MPNs, ET only affects megakaryopoiesis while erythropoiesis and granulopoeisis remain untouched [12]. Kaloutsi et al [13] conducted a study in 1991 to assess the degrees of megakaryopoiesis in the four classic MPNs. The group found a rate of 59.85 MKs/sq.mm in patients exhibiting ET. While significantly greater than the control rate of 19.7 MKs/sq.mm, this number was comparable to that of the other three diseases. The same group and others found that while clustering of MKs is present in ET, it is not substantial. The cells tend to be loosely distributed in the marrow or present in small groups close to sinus walls but not within their lumina [6,13,14].

Other Diagnostic Criteria and Clinical Manifestations

As the name of the disease implies, thrombocytosis is a crucial diagnostic criterion for ET. The theme of thrombocytosis will be present throughout this chapter as increased megakaryopoiesis tends to raise platelet counts. Platelet counts beyond 600×10^9/L (normal range is $150 - 400 \times 10^9$/L) are likely to be present in patients with ET.

As thrombocytosis may be a response to a condition such as an inflammatory disorder, hemorrhage, or infection [15,16], such a process must be ruled out.

Although the rise in platelet counts is a pathogenic mechanism, recent evidence shows that extreme thrombocytosis with platelet counts higher than 1000×10^9/L are actually associated with reduced rates of deleterious symptoms [17,18]. In distinguishing ET from other MPNs, the clinician should ensure that collagen fibrosis is absent from any bone marrow biopsy (unlike in primary myelofibrosis) [16].

The chief clinical manifestations in ET consist of both clotting events and hemorrhagic events.

The former include transient headaches, transient ischemic attacks, acroparesthesies, and and erythromelalgic symptoms which worsen in warm temperature and improve with cooler temperatures. Rarer but more severe clotting events may include deep vein thrombosis, pulmonary embolism, portal vein thrombosis, heart attack, and stroke. Although arterial thromboses are fairly common, venous thromboses have much lower incidences in ET than in other MPNs. Possible hemorrhagic events include easy bruising, epistaxis, gingival bleeding, uterine bleeding, and gastrointestinal tract bleeding. Splenomegaly and cyanosis can also occur as a result of hemorrhagic events [16,19]. Myelofibrosis may develop in patients with ET but is rare, occurring in approximately 2-6% of patients. Its risk increases when MK count is especially elevated [6,11].

Molecular Genetics

Excluding chronic myelogenous leukemia, the molecular events involved in the pathogenesis of MPNs have been poorly defined until recently. In 2005, multiple groups identified a gain-of-function mutation that was common to ET, primary myelofibrosis, and polycythemia vera. The V617F JAK2 mutation was shown to be an acquired mutation, being present in myeloid lineage cells but absent in T cells. The V617F JAK2 mutation exists in approximately 50% of ET patients [20-22].

Kravlovics et. al. postulate that the mutation gives hematopoietic precursor cells a proliferative advantage, thus leading to the MPN in affected patients [20].

Another group reports that ratio of mutant to wild-type JAK2 is crucial to the phenotype displayed by the patient [23]. These groups have found that the JAK2 mutation in ET can lead to more classic symptoms, longer duration of disease, more severe degrees of thrombocytosis, and more frequent rates of hemorrhage, fibrosis, and thrombosis. Mutations that affect c-mpl, the receptor for thrombopoietin, have also been discovered to be associated with ET. The W515L MPL and W515K MPL gain-of-function mutations are present in approximately 8% of cases [24,25].

Expression of these mutations increases JAK-STAT signaling, resulting in a myeloproliferative disease phenotype [26]. Recent studies by Klampfl et al. have identified mutations in the gene encoding calreticulin (CALR) in 67% of patients who have nonmutated V617F JAK2, W515L MPL, and W515K MPL essential thrombocythemia.

They also found that mutations in CALR are exclusive to essential thrombocythemia and primary myelofibrosis [27].

PRIMARY MYELOFIBROSIS

Histopathology

The distinguishing feature of MKs in Primary Myelofibrosis (PMF) is their considerable pleomorphy. Numerous groups report significant degrees of variance in the size of each MK, size of their nuclei, and morphology of their nuclei [7,8,28]. Generally, both the MKs and their nuclei are enlarged, although undersized abnormal MK elements may also be present [6,11]. A relatively unique feature of the nuclei is their unusual segmentation. Each nucleus has reduced levels of lobulation while multiple groups report that they display hypochromasia, leading to a characteristic bulbous or "cloud-like" appearance [6,29,30]. Adding to the pleomorphic nature of MKs in PMF are considerable alterations of their cytoplasmic and nuclear organization [12]. MK proliferation is another substantial feature of PMF. Kaloutsi et al report that MKs are more numerous in PMF than in all other chronic MPNs outside of chronic myelogenous leukemia with megakaryocytic increase. They report a cell count of 67.78 MKs/sq.mm compared to a control of 19.7 MKs/sq.mm. The same group reported MK clustering to be more prevalent in PMF than in the other classic MPNs [13]. Georgii et al. state that, unlike in ET, MK clustering in PMF tends to be around sinuses but contained within their lumina [6]. Although early stages of the disease display high levels of clustering, clustering may be reduced in frequency and in the number of MKs per cluster the latter stages of the disease [6,13]. In early stages of PMF, some of the hyperplastic and morphological characteristics of MKs may be confused with those in ET. However, the hyperplasia in ET is restricted to MKs, whereas both megakaryocytic and granulocytic proliferation is present in PMF. The proliferation of these two cell lines and lack of hyperplasia in the erythroid lineage leads to the histological finding of a relative decrease of erythroid precursors [12,31].

Outside of MKs, the main histological distinction of PMF is reticulin fibrosis. As with MKs, there are wide ranges of histological findings that may be seen regarding fibrosis, mainly owing to differences in stages of the disease. Early stages lack evidence of reticulin fibrosis, so the main diagnostic findings with respect to histology are the characteristic MKs along with granulocytic proliferation and a lack of erythroid proliferation – hence these stages are referred to as the "cellular phase" [32]. In latter stages, MK clustering is reduced and the main finding is reticulin fibrosis which may be complemented by collagen fibrosis – hence later stages are known as the "fibrotic phase" [11,32]. The peripheral blood smear can be an important diagnostic method, as PMF patients often display dacryocytosis (teardrop-shaped erythrocytes) and leukoerythroblastosis, which is an anemic condition characterized by immature granulocytes and nucleated erythrocytes [15,32].

Other Diagnostic Criteria and Clinical Manifestations

Beyond histology, other diagnostic criteria of PMF include elevated levels of LDH and thrombocytosis with platelets exceeding $400x10^9$/L. Anemia is another feature of the disease that varies by stages. While hemoglobin levels remain within the normal range in early stages, grade II anemia (8-10 g/dL Hb) manifests in intermediate stages of the disease and grade III anemia (<8 g/dL Hb) manifests in advanced stages [11,32]. Although some patients are asymptomatic at diagnosis, the majority display various levels of clinically evident signs and symptoms. More common manifestations are splenomegaly and hepatomegaly, while thrombotic events (especially venous thrombosis), hemorrhage, early satiety, pruritus, lymphadenopathy, ascites, and increased susceptibility to infection may also occur.

Enlargement of the spleen, liver, and lymph nodes occurs due to extramedullary hematopoesis that is characterisitic of myelofibrosis [32-34]. Osteosclerosis, present in 30-70% of patients, sets in during the fibrotic phase of the disease [32,33].

Molecular Genetics

The V617F JAK2 mutation has been identified as the mutation most closely associated with PMF, as multiple groups report its presence in approximately 50% of cases [20,35]. The same groups and others report that the presence of this mutation is linked to more classic symptoms, a higher incidence of thrombosis and hemorrhage, more platelets and MKs in the blood, and a longer duration of the disease [20,23,35]. A W515L MPL or W515K MPL gain of function mutation has been reported to be present in about 5% of cases [36].

The CALR mutation identified by Klampfl et al. was identified in 88% of patients with nonmutated JAK2 and MPL primary myclofibrosis [27]. While the GATA-1 gene has been speculated to be of importance in the pathogenesis of PMF, Vannucchi et al. report no evidence of GATA-1 mutations in patients.

However, the group did find that MKs from PMF patients have reduced GATA-1 content which may contribute to pathogenesis. They propose the gene as a novel disease marker for PMF [37].

POLYCYTHEMIA VERA

Histopathology

Similar to other MPNs, MKs and their nuclei in Polycythemia Vera (PV) are enlarged. Some studies report their size to be largest out of PV, ET, and PMF. A moderate degree pleomorphy exists in PV, and small to medium sized MKs may also be present in histological sections [7,8]. The MKs appear to lack any maturation abnormalities, and their nuclei are regularly lobulated and hyperchromatic. However, very late stages of the disease can present with a striking proliferation of anomalous MKs and fibrotic growths that can resemble PMF [11]. One of the primary diagnostic features of this disorder is the proliferation of all three major hematopoietic lineages (panmyelosis). However, the MK and erythroid lineages predominate [12]. The Kaloutsi et al study found MK proliferation to be similar to other classic MPNs at 59.59 MK/sq.mm. The same group reported that MK clustering does occur but the groups are loosely arranged [13]. These clusters are frequently localized toward the paratrabecular area and located around the sinuses but not in their lumina. The sinuses of the lumina frequently appear hyperplastic, and this is one of the key distinguishing features of PV [6,11]. Though PV is sometimes confused histologically with a reactive polycythemia, this can be avoided by looking for evidence of an inflammatory reaction with iron-filled macrophages and increased levels of plasma cells. This occurrence is common with reactive polycythemias but not PV [11,12].

Other Diagnostic Criteria and Clinical Manifestations

Measurement of erythropoietin (EPO) levels is recommended as a diagnostic tool for PV. The overabundance of erythroid cells actually leads to a lower concentration of EPO in the blood. Almost all PV patients exhibit EPO concentrations below the lower reference limit and one study found that 68% of patients in their cohort had undetectable levels of EPO [5]. Another study recommended utilizing c-mpl and polycythemia rubra vera-1 messenger RNA

(PRV-1 mRNA) as molecular markers for the disease. Although neither is considered to cause the disease, c-mpl is underexpressed and PRV-1 mRNA is overexpressed by PV patients [38]. One group reported that half of their set of PV patients possessed c-mpl levels that were absent or considerably decreased [39]. A separate group utilized qualitative reverse transcriptase PCR to determine that PRV-1 mRNA was the most common myeloproliferative marker found in their cohort of patients [40]. Although earlier studies have described increased red blood cell mass as a viable diagnostic tool [11], more recent studies have emphasized that this method is too expensive and unreliable be warranted for the diagnosis of PV [41,42].

The main clinical manifestations of PV include erythromelalgia, headaches, peripheral ischemia, and thrombotic events. Unlike in ET, the incidences of arterial and venous thrombotic events are approximately equal in PV. Other classic symptoms include pruritis, which occurs in roughly 40% of patients, and gouty arthritis, which is present in close to 20% of patients. PV patients may also present with hepatomegaly and prominent splenomegaly [5,14,16,19,43]. PV evolves to myelofibrosis in 10-15% of patients with high megakaryocytic involvement and increased LDH levels as risk factors for its development [6,44].

Molecular Genetics

The V617F JAK2 mutation is currently the only known mutation that is closely related to the pathogenesis of PV. One study found it to be present in over 80% of PV patients [22], while another group postulated the mutation to be present in virtually all patients [45]. An increased V617F JAK2 allele burden may serve as a risk factor for the development of post-PV myelofibrosis [44]. Patients with nonmutated V617 JAK2 were found to have lower platelet and leukocyte counts as compared to those with the V617 JAK2 mutation [46].

CHRONIC MYELOGENOUS LEUKEMIA

Histopathology

MKs in chronic myelogenous leukemia (CML) are especially distinct from those of the other three chronic MPNs. MKs along with their nuclei are actually reduced in size to roughly 80% of normal sizes. The cytoplasm is diminished, and nuclei display reduced segmentation and lobulation [7,8,47]. CML can be histologically subtyped into three different groups according to the numerical density of MKs: CML of common type, CML with megakaryocytic increase, and CML with megakaryocytic predominance. Georgii et al report the first type to comprise approximately 50-65% of patients, the second type to comprise 30-45%, and the last type to comprise roughly 5% [6]. The three types of the disease display vast differences with respect to MK numbers. The Kaloutsi et al study found CML of common type to have normal MK counts, reporting 15.54 MKs/sq.mm in histological sections compared to the control of 19.7 MKs/sq.mm. The group reported CML with megakaryocytic increase to display 69.91 MKs/sq.mm, which is a similar count to the other three classic MPNs. This study did not measure MK numbers for CML with megakaryocytic predominance, although the group did acknowledge the presence of this category of the disease [13]. Georgii et al defines CML with megakaryocytic predominance as over 70 MKs per sq mm. They also emphasize that this category of the disease is the only one in which MKs exhibit significant pleomorphic characteristics and gather into sheets of cells [6]. In all types of CML, the hematopoietic lineage that proliferates the most is the myeloid lineage. The primary histological finding is an excess of mature granulocytes along with their precursors [48]. The presence of Pseudo-Gaucher cells is also useful in diagnosis, as they are primarily restricted to cases of CML. These plasma cells closely resemble Gaucher cells, which are large and vacuolated cells with cytoplasm described as resembling crinkled paper. Psuedo-Gaucher cells are present in approximately 70% of patients, and numerical increases are correlated with more advanced stages of the disease with worse prognoses [49-51].

Other Diagnostic Criteria and Clinical Manifestations

As amplified granulopoiesis is a chief characteristic of CML, a complete blood count is very useful in diagnosis [48]. However, the diagnosis of the disease must ultimately be confirmed by cytogenetics or molecular testing, which is discussed later. CML can be divided into three stages based on symptoms and laboratory findings. The first phase is known as the chronic phase, and 85% of CML patients are in chronic phase at the time of diagnosis. Without treatment, the disease may progress to the accelerated phase and subsequently to blast crisis, the final stage. The chronic phase is largely asymptomatic. WHO criteria are commonly used to define the latter two stages. A patient is in the accelerated phase if one or more of the following criteria are present: myeloblasts comprising 10-19% of cells in the blood or marrow, greater than 20% basophils in the blood, thrombocytopenia (platelets below $100x10^9$/L) or thrombocytosis (platelets above $1000x10^9$/L), splenomegaly and elevated white blood cell count unresponsive to therapy, or evidence of cytogenic evolution. Blast crisis is defined as the presence of one or more of the following: myeloblasts comprise greater than 20% of cells in the blood or marrow, development of blasts outside the marrow, or bone marrow biopsy displaying sizeable clusters of blasts [52]. Blast crisis progresses similar to an acute leukemia and is characterized by short survival times [53]. Various groups have proposed phosphotyrosine or histamine levels as indicators of prognosis or the current stage of the disease [54,55]. More generalized symptoms of CML that may be present in any of the three phases include easy bruising, weight loss, anemia, hemorrhagic events, and gout [53,56,57]. The incidence of myelofibrosis during or after CML is approximately 20% [6].

Cytogenetics and Molecular Genetics

CML is chiefly characterized by a t(9;22)(q34;q11) translocation known as the Philadelphia chromosome. It is a translocation between chromsomes 9 and 22 that results in the BCR-ABL fusion gene [58-60]. Over 90% of CML patients test positive for the Philadelphia chromosome, usually by means of fluorescent in situ hybyridization or PCR detection of the fusion gene. Rarely, BCR-ABL fusion results from an atypical translocation. However, other diagnostic tests are also necessary because cytogenetic testing for the Philadelphia chromosome is not specific enough: it is also present in acute lympoblastic leukemia and acute myelogenous leukemia [53,58].

A small minority of CML patients test negative for the translocation. The molecular mechanism at work in some of these patients is currently unknown, and others may be affected by translocations whose outcomes represent a chronic leukemia that closely mimics CML. The most common of these other translocations are t(5;12)(q33;p13) and t(8;13)(p11;q12) [59,61,62].

TRANSIENT MYELOPROLIFERATIVE DISORDER / ACUTE MEGAKARYOBLASTIC LEUKEMIA

Histopathology

Transient myeloproliferative disorder (TMD) and acute megakaryoblastic leukemia (AMKL), as their names imply, are acute rather than chronic disorders. AMKL is a more severe disease, and it can evolve from certain cases of TMD. Both disorders exhibit decreased leukocyte counts and proliferation of the megakaryocytic lineage. Although the Kaloutsi et al study evaluated only the classic MPNs and not these two diseases, it is known that cells of the MK lineage in these two disorders are increased to the point at which they crowd out and suppress other hematopoietic lineages [4]. However, these diseases are rarely confused with the MPNs as TMD and AMKL primarily manifest in infants while the MPNs manifest in adults. While the other diseases in this chapter have been characterized by increases in mature MKs, TMD and AMKL are characterized by a proliferation of megakaryoblasts, their precursors. In histological examinations these blasts exhibit a unique morphology, frequently displaying surface blebs, clumping, and binulceation. They are medium to large sized and exhibit a high nuclear to cytoplasmic ratio. Megakaryoblasts are structurally and immunologically similar in both disorders, but a greater than 30% incidence of blast cells in the marrow confirms a diagnosis of AMKL [4,52,63].

Other Diagnostic Criteria and Clinical Manifestations

Athale et al conducted a study examining the various characteristics of AMKL and found two to be highly diagnostic for the disease. The first is the unique morphology of megakaryoblasts as described above.

The second, detected by immunohistochemical methods, is that the blasts exhibit alpha naphthyl acetate esterase activity that is partially inhibited by sodium fluoride [63].

Other characteristics of the blasts include staining negatively with Sudan black B and a lack of myeloperoxidase activity [4].

Clinical manifestations vary considerably between different cases of TMD. Some patients are asymptomatic while on the other end of the spectrum are patients with thrombocytopenia, respiratory problems, hepatomegaly, liver dysfunction, and easy bruising. Fatalities, while rare, can occur if hepatic fibrosis develops and MKs infiltrate the liver [4,64,65]. In a study conducted by the Children's Oncology Group on 48 infants with TMD and Down syndrome, early death transpired in 17% and leukemia developed in another 19%. Early death was correlated with an elevated white blood cell count at diagnosis along with increased levels of liver enzymes and bilirubin [65].

TMD progresses to AMKL in 20-30% of cases [4,65]. Organomegaly is a prominent symptom of the disease. One study identified hepatomegaly in roughly half of their patient cohort as well as splenomegaly in 39% and lymphadenopathy in 29% [63]. Bone marrow aspirates from some AMKL patients have been shown to display myelofibrosis [4]. The Athale et al study identified a moderate to severe escalation in reticulin fibrosis in almost half of patients that were examined [63].

Molecular Genetics

TMD and AMKL are closely associated with GATA-1, a transcription factor that plays a crucial role in the MK, erythroid, mast cell, and eosinophil hematopoietic cell lines.

In these diseases, a somatic mutation involves a splice in exon 2 of GATA-1 that leads to the creation of GATA-1s, which is a shorter isoform of the gene. The mutation is strongly linked to trisomy 21, shown by the fact that children with Down syndrome are up to 500 times more likely to acquire AMKL. Nonetheless, patients with AMKL associated with trisomy 21 have better prognosis than other AMKL patients [4,63]. The Athale et al study reported drastically lower 5-year survival rates in the de novo form of the disease. The group also reported that while the frequency of myelofibrosis appeared to be the same between de novo AMKL and AMKL associated with trisomy 21, de novo AMKL tended to have more severe degrees of fibrosis [63]. The t(1;22)(p13;q13) chromosomal translocation is also linked to AMKL. Approximately 30% of cases are associated with this translocation rather than trisomy 21 [66].

CONCLUSION

Excepting of certain cases of CML, the four MPNs that enhance megakaryopoeisis tend to exhibit the same amount of MK proliferation.

Hence, they are best distinguished histologically by MK morphology or the presence or absence of the proliferation of other hematopoietic lineages. The presence of reticulin fibrosis can be a useful diagnostic tool, but there are pitfalls to this as early stages of PMF do not display fibrotic tissue and later stages of the other MPNs have the potential to develop myelofibrosis. It remains difficult to distinguish the diseases based on clinically evident symptoms.

Thrombocytosis, organomegaly, clotting events, and hemorrhagic events are themes that remain fairly constant through the four MPNs covered by this paper. Likewise, testing for the presence of the V617F JAK2 mutation can help to diagnose ET, PMF, or PV but cannot distinguish between the three disorders. However, recent studies identifying the CALR mutation suggest its presence could be used to distinguish ET and PMF from PV. A positive test for the Philadelphia chromosome strongly indicates CML though histological and other diagnostic methods are necessary to confirm the diagnosis. AMKL diagnosis requires an approach that involves both histopathology and immunohistochemistry, although there are strong clinical indicators. In summary, while it is clear that an array of laboratory and clinical information is advised to diagnose an MPN, bone marrow histology may result in the most discerning data.

ACKNOWLEDGMENTS

This work was supported by the Indiana - Clinical and Translational Sciences Institute funded, in part by NIH grants RR025760 and RR025761 (MAK), the Summer Research Program in Academic Medicine, Indiana University School of Medicine, funded in part by NIH grant HL110854 (MAK, SMB), the Department of Orthopaedic Surgery, Indiana University School of Medicine (MAK, CS, PDM), and by NIH grants NIAMS R03 AR055269 (MAK), NIAMS R01 AR060332 (MAK), and NIA R01 AG046246 (MAK).

REFERENCES

[1]   Dameshek W. Some speculations on the myeloproliferative syndromes. *Blood 1951*;6:372-5.

[2]   Tefferi A, Vardiman JW. Classification and diagnosis of myeloproliferative neoplasms: The 2008 world health organization criteria and point-of-care diagnostic algorithms. *Leukemia* 2008;22:14-22.

[3]   Tefferi A, Thiele J, Vardiman JW. The 2008 world health organization classification system for myeloproliferative neoplasms: Order out of chaos. *Cancer* 2009;115:3842-7.

[4]   Ciovacco WA, Raskind WH, Kacena MA. Human phenotypes associated with GATA-1 mutations. *Gene* 2008;427:1-6.

[5]   Johansson P, Safai-Kutti S, Lindstedt G, Suurkula M, Kutti J. Red cell mass, spleen size and plasma erythropoietin in polycythaemia vera and apparent polycythaemia. *Acta. Haematologica* 2002;108:1-7.

[6]   Georgii A, Buesche G, Kreft A. The histopathology of chronic myeloproliferative diseases. *Baillieres Clin. Haematol.* 1998;11:724-49.

[7]   Nafe R, Georgii A, Kaloutsi V, Fritsch RS, Choritz H. Planimetric analysis of megakaryocytes and the four main groups of chronic myeloproliferative disorders. *Virchows Archive B* 1991;61:111-6.

[8]   Nafe R, Kaloutsi V, Fritsch RS, Georgii A. Quantitative cytomorphology of megakaryocytes in chronic myeloproliferative disorders--analysis of planimetric and numeric characteristics by means of a knowledge based system. *Exp. Pathol.* 1990;40:213-9.

[9]   Thiele J, Schneider G, Hoeppner B, Wienhold S, Zankovich R, Fischer R. Histomorphometry of bone marrow biopsies in chronic myeloproliferative disorders with associated thrombocytosis – features of significance for the diagnosis of primary (essential) thrombocythaemia. Virchows *Arch. A Pathol. Anat. Histopathol.* 1988;413:407-17.

[10]   Georgii A, Buhr T, Buesche G, Kreft A, Choritz H. Classification and staging of ph-negative myeloproliferative disorders by histopathology from bone marrow biopsies. *Leuk. Lymphoma* 1996;22:15-29.

[11]   Michiels JJ, Thiele J. Clinical and pathological criteria for the diagnosis of essential thrombocythemia, polycythemia vera, and idiopathic myelofibrosis (agnogenic myeloid metaplasia). *Int. J. Hematol.* 2002;76:133-45.

[12]   Thiele J, Kvasnicka HM, Vardiman J. Bone marrow histopathology in the diagnosis of chronic myeloproliferative disorders: A forgotten pearl. *Best Pract. Res. Clin. Haematol.* 2006;19:413-37.

[13]   Kaloutsi V, Fritsch RS, Buhr T, Restrepo-Specht I, Widjaja W, Georgii A. Megakaryocytes in chronic myeloproliferative disorders: Numerical

density correlated between different entities. *Virchows Arch. A. Pathol. Anat Histopathol* 1991;418:493-7.

[14] Michiels J. Erythromelalgia and vascular complications in polycythemia vera. *Semin. Thromb. Hemost* 1997;23:441-54.

[15] Tefferi A, Thiele J, Orazi A, et al. Proposals and rationale for the revision of the world health organization diagnostic criteria for polycythemia vera, essential thrombocythemia, and primary myelofibrosis: Recommendations from an ad hoc international expert panel. *Blood* 2007;110:1092-7.

[16] Andersson BS. Essential thrombocythemia: Diagnosis and treatment; with special emphasis on the use of anagrelide. *Hematology* 2002;7: 173-7.

[17] Carobbio A, Finazzi G, Antonioli E, et al. Thrombocytosis and leukocytosis interaction in vascular complications of essential thrombocythemia. *Blood* 2008;112:3135-7.

[18] Tefferi A. Platelet count in essential thrombocythemia: The more the better? *Blood* 2008;112:3526.

[19] van Genderen PJ, Michiels JJ. Erythromelalgia: A pathognomonic microvascular thrombotic complication in essential thrombocythemia and polycythemia vera. *Semin. Thromb. Hemost.* 1997;23:357-63.

[20] Kralovics R, Passamonti F, Buser AS, et al. A gain-of-function mutation of JAK2 in myeloproliferative disorders. *N. Engl. J. Med.* 2005;352:1779-90.

[21] McLornan D, Percy M, McMullin MF. JAK2 V617F: A single mutation in the myeloproliferative group of disorders. *Ulster. Med. J.* 2006;75:112-9.

[22] James C, Ugo V, Le Couédic JP, et al. A unique clonal JAK2 mutation leading to constitutive signaling causes polycythaemia vera. *Nature* 2005;434:1144-8.

[23] Tiedt R, Hao-Shen H, Sobas MA, et al. Ratio of mutant JAK2-V617F to wild-type Jak2 determines the MPD phenotypes in transgenic mice. *Blood* 2008;111:3931-40.

[24] Pardanani AD, Levine RL, Lasho T, et al. MPL515 mutations in myeloproliferative and other myeloid disorders: A study of 1182 patients. *Blood* 2006;108:3472-6.

[25] Beer PA, Campbell PJ, Scott LM, et al. MPL mutations in myeloproliferative disorders: Analysis of the PT-1 cohort. *Blood* 2008;112:141-9.

[26] Levine RL. Another piece of the myeloproliferative neoplasms puzzle. *N Engl J Med* 2013;369:2451-2.

[27] Klampfl T, Gisslinger H, Harutyunyan A. Somatic mutations of calreticulin in myeloproliferative neoplasms. *N. Engl. J. Med.* 2013;369:2379-90.

[28] Ciurea SO, Merchant D, Mahmud N, et al. Pivotal contributions of megakaryocytes to the biology of idiopathic myelofibrosis. *Blood* 2007;110:986-93.

[29] Buhr T, Choritz H, Georgii A. The impact of megakaryocyte proliferation for the evolutionof myelofibrosis. histological follow-up study in 186 patients with chronic myeloid leukaemia. *Virchows Arch. A. Pathol. Anat. Histopathol.* 1992;420:473-8.

[30] Buhr T, Georgii A, Choritz H. Myelofibrosis in chronic myeloproliferative disorders: Incidence among subtypes according to the hannover classification. *Pathol. Res. Pract.* 1993;189:121-32.

[31] Thiele J, Kvasnicka HM. A critical reappraisal of the WHO classification of the chronic myeloproliferative disorders. *Leuk. Lymphoma* 2006;47:381-96.

[32] Tefferi A. Primary myelofibrosis. *Cancer Treat Res.* 2008;142:29-49.

[33] Ward HP, Block MH. The natural history of agnogenic myeloid metaplasia and a critical evaluation of its relationship with the myeloid proliferative disorders. *Medicine* 1971;50:357-420.

[34] Cervantes F, Alvarez-Larrán A, Arellano-Rodrigo E, Granell M, Domingo A, Montserrat E. Frequency and risk factors for thrombosis in idiopathic myelofibrosis: Analysis in a series of 155 patients from a single institution. *Leukemia* 2006;20:55-60.

[35] Li WD, Li JY, Zhang SJ, Qiu HR, Xu W, Wang JS. JAK2V617F mutation in patients with idiopathic myelofibrosis. *Zhongguo Shi Yan Xue Ye Xue Za Zhi* 2007;15:387-90.

[36] Pikman Y, Lee BH, Mercher T, et al. MPLW515L is a novel somatic activating mutation in myelofibrosis with myeloid metaplasia. *PLoS Med* 2006;3:e270.

[37] Vannucchi AM, Pancrazzi A, Guglielmelli P, et al. Abnormalities of GATA-1 in megakaryocytes from patients with idiopathic myelofibrosis. *American Journal of Pathology* 2005;167:849-58.

[38] Pahl HL. Diagnostic approaches to polycythemia vera in 2004. *Expert Review of Molecular Diagnostics 2004*;4:495-502.

[39] Le Blanc K, Andersson P, Samuelsson J. Marked heterogeneity in protein levels and functional integrity of the thrombopoietin receptor c-

mpl in polycythaemia vera. *British Journal of Haematology* 2000;108:80-5.

[40] Teofili L, Giona F. Martini M, Cenci T. Guidi F, et al. Markers of myeloproliferative diseases in childhood polycythemia vera and essential thrombocythemia. *Journal of Clinical Oncology* 2007;25:1048-53.

[41] Tefferi A. The rise and fall of red cell mass measurement in polycythemia vera. *Current Hematology Reports* 2005;4:213-7.

[42] Sirhan S, Fairbanks VF, Tefferi A. Red cell mass and plasma volume measurements in polycythemia: Evaluation of performance and practical utility. *Cancer* 2005;104:213-5.

[43] Berlin NI. Diagnosis and classification of polycythemias. *Semin Hematol* 1975;12:339-51.

[44] Alvarez-Larran A, Bellosillo B, Martinez-Aviles L, et al. Postpolycythaemic myelofibrosis: Frequency and risk factors for this complication in 116 patients. *British Journal of Haematology* 2009;146:504-9.

[45] Verstovsek S, Silver RT, Cross NC, Tefferi A. JAK2V617F mutational frequency in polycythemia vera: 100%; >90%; less? *Leukemia* 2006;20:2067.

[46] Caires dos Santos L, Correa da Costa Ribeiro J, Silva N, et al. Cytogenetics, JAK2 and MPL mutations in polycythemia vera, primary myelofibrosis and essential thrombocythemia. *Rev. Bras. Hematol.* Hemoter 2011;33:417-24.

[47] Thiele J, Fischer R. Megakaryocytopoiesis in haematological disorders: Diagnostic featuresof bone marrow biopsies. *Virchows Archive A* 1991;418:87-97.

[48] Hehlmann R, Hochhaus A, Baccarani M, European LeukemiaNet. Chronic myeloid leukaemia. *Lancet* 2007;370:342-50.

[49] Buesche G, Schlue J, Majewski H. Numerical increase of pseudo-gaucher cells in CML indication of a more advanced stage of disease. *Blood* 1995;86:3151.

[50] Buesche G, Majewski H, Schlue J, et al. Frequency of pseudo-gaucher cells within diagnostic bone marrow biopsies from patients with a ph-positive CML. *Virchows Arch.* 1997;430:139-48.

[51] Ross DJ, Spira S, Buchbinder N. Gaucher cells in pulmonary-capillary blood in association with pulmonary hypertension. *N. Engl. J. Med.* 1997;336:379-81.

[52] Vardiman J, Harris N, Brunning R. The world health organization (WHO) classification of the myeloid neoplasms. *Blood* 2002;100:2292-302.

[53] Tefferi A. Classification; diagnosis and management of myeloproliferative disorders in the JAK2V617F era. *Hematology Am Soc Hematol Educ Program* 2006;:240-5.

[54] Sun X, Li J, Chen J, et al. Flow cytometric assay of phosphotyrosine levels in bcr-abl-positive chronic myelogenous leukemias: A potential prognostic marker. *Annals of Hematology* 2009;88:29-36.

[55] Agis H, Sperr WR, Herndlhofer S, et al. Clinical and prognostic significance of histamine monitoring in patients with CML during treatment with imatinib (STI571). *Ann. Oncol.* 2007;18:843-1.

[56] Savage DG, Szydlo RM, Goldman JM. Clinical features at diagnosis in 430 patients with chronic myeloid leukaemia seen at a referral centre over a 16-year period. *Br. J. Haematol.* 1997;96:111-6.

[57] Faderl S, Talpaz M, Estrov Z, Kantarjian HM. Chronic myelogenous leukemia: Biology and therapy. *Ann. Intern. Med.* 1999;131:207-19.

[58] Kurzrock R, Kantarjian HM, Druker BJ, Talpaz M. Philadelphia chromosome-positive leukemias: From basic mechanisms to molecular therapeutics. *Ann. Intern. Med.* 2003;138:819-30.

[59] Goldman JM, Melo JV. Chronic myeloid leukemia – advances in biology and new approaches to treatment. *N. Engl. J. Med.* 2003;349:1451-64.

[60] Faderl S, Talpaz M, Estrov Z, Kantarjian HM. Chronic myelogenous leukemia: Biology and therapy, *Annals of Internal Medicine* 1999;131:207-19.

[61] Golub TR, Barker GF, Lovett M, Gilliland DG. Fusion of PDGF receptor beta to a novel ets-like gene; tel; in chronic myelomonocytic leukemia with t(5;12) chromosomal translocation. *Cell* 1994;77:307-16.

[62] Reiter A, Sohal J, Kulkarni S, et al. Consistent fusion of ZNF198 to the fibroblast growth factor receptor-1 in the t(8;13)(p11;q12) myeloproliferative syndrome. *Blood* 1998;92:1735-42.

[63] Athale UH, Razzouk BI, Raimondi SC, et al. Biology and outcome of childhood acute megakaryoblastic keukemia: A single institution's experience. *Blood* 2001;97:3727-32.

[64] Massey GV. Transient leukemia in newborns with down syndrome. *Pediatr. Blood Cancer* 2005;44:29-32.

[65] Massey GV, Zipursky A, Chang MN, et al. A prospective study of the natural history of transient leukemia (TL) in neonates with down syndrome (DS): Children's oncology group (COG) study POG-9481. *Blood* 2006;107:4606-13.

[66] Lion T, Haas OA. Acute megakaryocytic leukemia with the t(1;22)(p13;q13). *Leuk. Lymphoma* 1993;11:15-20.

In: Myeloproliferative Disorders
Editor: Anthony M. Camden

ISBN: 978-1-63321-201-5
© 2014 Nova Science Publishers, Inc.

Chapter 3

PCM1-JAK2 MYELODYSPLASTIC/ MYELOPROLIFERATIVE NEOPLASMS

Elena Masselli[1,2], Marco Vitale[2] and Franco Aversa[1]*
[1]Clinical and Experimental Medicine, Unit of Hematology, University of Parma, Italy
[2]Biological, Biotechnological and Translational Sciences, Unit of Human Anatomy and Histology, University of Parma, Italy

ABSTRACT

Janus-activated kinase 2 *(JAK2)* translocations have been described in hematologic malignancies involving both lymphoid and myeloid lineages. Better characterized translocation partners are *ETV6/TEL* on chromosome 12, *BCR* on chromosome 22 and the autoantigen Pericentriolar material-1 *(PCM1)* on chromosome 8. *PCM1-JAK2* fusion events are extremely rare and, to our best knowledge, less than 30 clinical cases have been reported so far in the literature. Although the clinical onset of these disorders is extremely heterogeneous, several cases present with a myelodysplastic/ myeloproliferative disease with striking dysplastic features of the erythroid compartment.

---

* Corresponding author: Franco Aversa, MD, Clinical and Experimental Medicine, Unit of Hematology, University of Parma, Via Gramsci n.14, 43126 Italy. Tel: +39 0521 033272 Fax: +39 0521 033264 Email: franco.aversa@unipr.it.

Although recent studies showed an activation of the JAK/STAT axis in a *PCM1-JAK2*-transformed murine fibroblast or human lymphoma cell lines, little is known about signaling in primary cells from *PCM1-JAK2* patients. This aspect is extremely relevant if we consider the availability of new drugs targeting the JAK/STAT pathway (i.e. ruxolitinib).

Our group has recently studied the signaling pathways potentially activated by the PCM1-JAK2 chimeric protein in a patient harboring the rare translocation t(8;9)(p22;24), demonstrating that the ERK1/2 pathway is the signaling cascade primarily activated in *PCM1-JAK2* patient's neoplastic cells.

In this chapter, we will review the main aspects of *PCM1-JAK2*-related myeloid malignancies focusing on the newest biological insights and their implication for therapy.

INTRODUCTION

Since the discovery, by Nowell and Hungerford in 1960 [1], that a chromosomal abnormality - subsequently identified as a balanced reciprocal translocation between the long arms of chromosome 9 and chromosome 22, t(9;22)(q34;q11.2)/*BCR-ABL1* [2] - was responsible for a clinical entity named chronic myeloid leukemia (CML), many advances have been done in the field of cytogenetic alterations in hematologic neoplasms.

This concept is well represented by the spirit of the revised World Health Organization (WHO) classification of myeloid neoplasms [3], which confers an outstanding relevance to cytogenetic abnormalities, identified as mandatory diagnostic tools and essential prognostic indicators.

The t(9;22)(q34;q11.2)/*BCR-ABL1* paved the way for the discovery of a series of translocations involving various tyrosine kinase (TK) genes other than *ABL1*, such as *PDGFRA, PDGFRB, FGFR* and *JAK2*. These cytogenetic abnormalities represent a pathogenetic hallmark of myeloproliferative disorders (MPNs) and lead to the constitutive activation of TKs or TK-dependent pathways [4].

Indeed, myeloproliferative disorders associated with translocation of *PDGFRA, PDGFRB. FGFR1* (i.e. *FIP1L1-PDGFRA, ETV6-PDGFRB* and *ZNF198-FGFR*) represent a defined and separate subtype of myeloid and lymphoid neoplasms according to the WHO 2008 classification [3].

Fusion Genes Involving *JAK2*

Translocations involving *JAK2* occur at a significant lower frequency than fusions involving *ABL1* or growth factor receptors (*PDGFRA, PDGFRB, FGFR1*). As pointed out by Walz et al., while on one side the clinical phenotype of JAK2 fusion-related hematologic malignancies closely recalls Philadelphia-positive CML (onset as chronic phase and then progression to an accelerated and, eventually, blast phase) than JAK2-mutated classic MPNs (i.e. PV, ET and PMF), on the other hand it appears to be characterized by a more aggressive course and unfavorable outcome than typical CML [4].

JAK2 fusion gene-related hematologic neoplasms are very rare diseases. In this contest, pericentriolar material 1 *(PCM1)* is the most frequent partner gene of *JAK2*. However, other partner genes have been reported in the literature such as *ETV6, BCR1, PAX5, SSBP2* and *SEC31A. ETV6-JAK2* fusion gene arises as a consequence of t(9;12) or variant translocations and, so far, it has been described in cases presenting with a chronic MPD or pre-B/T acute lymphoblastic leukemia (ALL) [5-6]. *BCR-JAK2* fusion, deriving from t(9;22), has been associated with atypical CML, acute myeloid leukemia (AML) and B cell-ALL [7-8]. Translocations involving *PAX5* and *SSBP2* (Single Stranded Binding Protein 2) have been recently published as single-case reports manifesting as childhood ALL and pre-B ALL, respectively [9-10].

It is clear from this list that JAK2 fusion gene-related disorders occur in both lymphoid and myeloid hematologic malignancies without marked lineage preference. This is valid also for t(8;9)/*PCM1-JAK2* related diseases, on which we will focus in the present chapter.

NORMAL STRUCTURE AND FUNCTION OF PCM1 AND JAK2

PCM1

The *PCM1* gene is located on chromosome band 8p22-p21.3 and encodes for a 228-kDa centrosomal protein containing multiple coiled-coil motifs that is ubiquitously expressed in mammalian tissues.

The centrosome is responsible for microtubule organization, which, in turns, is essential for multiple cell function such as directional intracellular transport, cell shape and motility and the formation of the spindle apparatus during cell division [11]. The centrosome consists of two centriolar cilinders surrounded by an osmiophilic cloud of electron-dense matrix made of various proteins (pericentrin, ninein and centrin), the so called pericentriolar material [12-14]. The pericentriolar material is a very dynamic structure, capable to exchange proteins with the cell cytoplasm thanks to the pericentriolar satellites, non membranous granules with a diameter of 70-100 nm [15]. The first identified molecular component of pericentriolar satellites is PCM1.

The role of PCM1 and pericentriolar satellites remained scantly characterized for decades, till Balczon et al., in 1994, described for first a distinct cell-cycle dependent interaction of PCM1 with the centrosome complex, regulated in a timely-specific manner (association during G1, S and early G2 phases; dissociation during late G2 phase, when the cell prepare for mitosis) [16].

Few years later, Dammermann et al. in 2002 and Hames et al. 2005 defined PCM1 functions. Specifically, they demonstrated that PCM1 is critical for the correct assembly of the centrosome - mediating the transport of its components from the cytoplasm to the centrosome along microtubules via dynein motor complexes - and for the organization of a radial microtubule network that is critical for cell division. The disruption of PCM1 function leads to improper functioning of pericentriolar satellites and consequent impaired protein integration to the centrosome and loss of microtubule organization [11, 17]. Finally, the role of PCM1 in the regulation of cell cycle, has been elegantly described by Balczon et al., who demonstrated, by injecting anti-PCM1 antibodies into murine fertilized zygotes, that PCM1 is essential for completion of interphase and for cell cycle progression [18].

Interestingly, as observed by Reiter et al. [19], PCM1 is not the sole centrosomal protein that is involved in hematologic neoplasms. In fact, the gene encoding for ninein *(NIN),* located on chromosome 14, has been shown to fuse to *PDGFRB* in a Imatinib-responsive chronic myeloproliferative syndrome [20]. Additionally, *FOP* (FGFR1 oncogene partner) on chromosome 6 and *CEP1* (also known as *CNTRL* or *CEP110*) on chromosome 9 are fused with *FGFR1* in the 8p11 myeloproliferative syndromes, resulting in t(6;8) and t(8;9) translocations.

The reason why centrosomal proteins are relatively frequent translocation partners of genes encoding for tyrosin kinases is not clear; a possible explanation could be found in their ubiquitous expression and in the fact they contain self-association motifs.

Implication of PCM1 in non-hematologic malignancies has been described by Corvi et al. in a case of thyroid papillary carcinoma characterized by t(8;10)(p22;q11) leading to PCM1-RET fusion [21].

JAK2

JAK2 is a member of a protein family encompassing four structural tightly related TKs: JAK1, JAK2, JAK3 and non-receptor tyrosine protein kinase 2 (TYK2), named after the two-faced Roman god Janus because of their symmetric structure.

The *JAK2* gene maps on chromosome band 9p24 and its activity is required for signaling to the cytoplasm by type I and type II cytokine receptors that lack intrinsic TK activity. The majority of cytokine receptors modulating the activity of hematopoietic stem- and progenitor-cells belongs to the type I cytokine receptor family, while type II cytokine receptors are primarily bound by interferon. Overall, these non-receptor TKs play a crucial role in multiple intracellular signaling pathways that modulate cell proliferation, differentiation, survival and apoptosis.

JAK2 structure is composed of seven domains (JH1-7); the JH1 domain is located at the carboxyl-terminus and is provided with TK activity. The JH2 moiety, or pseudokinase domain, is catalytically inactive and regulates the JH1 kinase domain activity in a negative fashion. JH3–JH4 domains shares homology with Src homology 2 (SH2) domains. The amino terminal domain (JH4–JH7) is known as the FERM (short for 4.1 protein, Ezrin, Radixin and Moesin) domain, which engages with cytokine receptors. Upon ligand binding, JAK2 undergoes to conformational changes that abrogate the inhibition of JH1 by JH2, allowing JAK2 phosphorylation and dimerization. Once activated, JAK2 is capable to bind to the SH2 domain of intracellular downstream molecules that, in turns, trigger the activation of a cascade of signaling pathways deeply interconnected and represented by:

- Signal Transducers and Activators of Transcription (STAT pathway);
- Ras-Raf-Mitogen Activated Protein Kinase (MAPK)/ Extracellular signaling-Related Kinase (ERK) (Ras-Raf-MEK-ERK) pathway;
- Phoshatidylinositol 3-Kinase (PI3-K)/PDK1/Akt pathway;
- Phospholipase C (PLC) γ pathway.

As a result, the final target of each signaling cascade undergoes phosphorylation, activation, rapid nuclear translocation where it binds to specific DNA sequences and activates transcription [22].

Recent data support the new concept the JAK2 itself is capable to migrate into the nucleus, where it modulates directly gene expression via chromatin remodeling. In fact, JAK2 phosphorylates histone H3 at tyrosine 41 (H3Y41), disrupting the binding of the transcriptional repressor heterochromatin protein 1α (HP1α) from chromatin and leading to aberrant gene expression, genome instability and oncogenesis [23].

JAK2 is deregulated in hematologic malignancies by copy number alterations, mutations and chromosomal translocations. The most common mechanism of activation of JAK2 is represented by the well-known V617F gain-of-function mutation in exon 14, described by three different groups in 2005 in approximately 95% of patients affected by polycythemia vera (PV) and 50% of patients with essential thrombocythemia (ET) and primary myelofibrosis (PMF). It is also present in 5-15% of patients with myelodysplastic/myeloprolifeative syndromes and ~50% of patients affected by refractory anemia with ringed sideroblasts and thrombocythosis (RARS-t) [24-26].

Finally, other activating mutations located in exon 12 of JAK2 (base pair substitutions, deletions, insertions and duplications) have been described in a small percentage of patients (3-5%) who fulfill the WHO criteria for PV but are *JAK2*V617F negative [27].

The effects of JAK2 activation are ligand-independent activation, cytokine-hypersensitivity, neoplastic transformation and abnormal cell proliferation.

PCM1-JAK2-RELATED NEOPLASMS

Clinical Presentation and Histopathological Features

PCM1-JAK2-related hematologic malignancies are extremely rare. So far, only 27 cases have been published in the literature [19, 28-38]. All these cases have been summarized in Table 1, stating from the first reports by Reiter and colleagues in 2005 [19] till the most recent one by Masselli et al. in 2013 [34].

Young adults are affected more than elderly (one third of the patients has ≤ 50 years, with a median age of 47 years, ranging from 12 to 75 years), although a few cases of people aged over 70 have been described, almost all in the last year (6 in total, cases n. 3, 6, 18, 19, 20 and 21) [19, 33, 36]. A striking male predominance can be seen (85.2%). The reasons of this gender skewing are unknown.

Clinical presentation is extremely variable since the disease may hit both the myeloid and the lymphoid lineage. Overall, 7 patients presented with atypical chronic myeloid leukemia (aCML), 6 patients with AML, 4 patients with chronic eosinophilic leukemia - not otherwise specified (CEL-NOS), 3 patients with an unclassifiable myelodysplastic/myeloproliferative neoplasm, 2 patients with an unclassifiable myeloproliferative neoplasm, 2 patients with de-novo acute lymphoblastic leukemia, 1 T-cell lymphoma and 1 erythroid leukemia.

Thus, although both hematopoietic lineages are affected, the great majority of the patients presented with a chronic or acute myeloid neoplasms (23 out of 27 patients, 85.2%) since only 4 patients were affected by a lymphoid malignancy (cases n. 4, 7, 15 and 24)[19, 28, 36]. Interestingly, 3 of these cases represented a lymphoid blast crisis of a chronic myeloid disorder (cases n. 4, 7 and 24) [19, 36].

The most common clinical onset is represented by a chronic myeloproliferative (MPN) or myelodysplastic/myeloproliferative disorders (MDS/MPN) and, specifically, aCML is the most frequent category. Patients presented with the typical stigmata of a chronic MPN such as left-shift leukocytosis, splenomegaly, variable degree of bone marrow fibrosis and anemia.

Acute leukemia (AL) may represent the evolution of a chronic myeloproliferative or, less frequently, lymphoproliferative disorder - which mirrors the blast phase in *BCR-ABL*-positive CML (case n. 1, 3, 7, 14 and 24) [19, 29, 36] - or a *de novo* disease, as described in patients n. 4, 16, 19, 20 and 23 [19, 32, 36].

Eosinophilia is a dominant, recurrent feature. Four cases were diagnosed with a CEL-NOS, and one third of the other 23 patients presented bone marrow hyperplasia of the eosinophilic lineage frequently associated to increased eosinophil count also in the peripheral blood. Bone marrow fibrosis is also a common feature, described in 6 out 27 cases (22.2%).

Table 1. Cases associated with *PCM1-JAK2* fusion reported so far in the literature

Case n.	Ref.	Age (y)	Gender	Diagnosis	Cytogenetics	FISH	RT-PCR	Therapy	Achievement of CyR	Achievement of MolR	Peculiar features
1	Reiter et al.	54	M	AML	t(8;9) (p23;p24)	*JAK2:* RP11-3H3 and RP11-28A9; *PCM1:* RP11-49F3 and RP11-3K23	No	intensive CHT INF	No	ND	myelofibrosis
2	Reiter et al.	47	M	CEL	t(8;9) (p22;p23)	*JAK2:* RP11-3H3 and RP11-28A9; *PCM1:* RP11-49F3 and RP11-3K23	*PCM1:* exon 35; *JAK2:* exon 9	INF	Yes (CCyR)	ND	myelofibrosis Eosinophilia
3	Reiter et al.	74	M	aCML	t(8;9) (p22;p24)	*JAK2:* RP11-3H3 and RP11-28A9; *PCM1:* RP11-49F3 and RP11-3K23	*PCM1:* exon 25; *JAK2:* exon 9	watch and wait	No	ND	eosinophilia progression to AL
4	Reiter et al.	50	M	Pre-B ALL	t(8;9) (p21;p24)	*JAK2:* RP11-3H3 and RP11-28A9; *PCM1:* RP11-49F3 and RP11-3K23	*PCM1:* exon 35; *JAK2:* exon 9	intensive CHT	No	ND	death during induction CHT
5	Reiter et al.	42	M	aCML	t(8;9) (p21;p24)	*JAK2:* RP11-3H3 and RP11-28A9; *PCM1:* RP11-49F3 and RP11-3K23	*PCM1:* exon 35; *JAK2:* exon 9	allo-BMT	ND	ND	eosinophilia
6	Reiter et al.	72	M	aCML	t(8;9) (p22;p23) ins(1;1) (p34;p36p34)	*JAK2:* RP11-3H3 and RP11-28A9; *PCM1:* RP11-49F3 and RP11-3K23	*PCM1:* exon 35; *JAK2:* exon 9	-	No	ND	death within 96h after admission

Case n.	Ref.	Age (y)	Gender	Diagnosis	Cytogenetics	FISH	RT-PCR	Therapy	Achievment of CyR	Achievment of MoIR	Peculiar features
7	Reiter et al.	32	M	aCML→ALL	t(8;9)(p21;p24)	*JAK2:* RP11-3H3 and RP11-28A9; *PCM1:* RP11-49F3 and RP11-3K23	*PCM1:* exon 28; *JAK2:* exon 9	allo-BMT	ND	ND	lymphoid blast crisis
8	Murati et al.	45	M	Atypical MPN	t(8;9)(p22;p24)	*JAK2:* RP11-927H16 *PCM1:* RP11-484L21	No	HU, INF, imatinib	No	ND	progressive disease
9	Murati et al.	12	F	EL	t(8;9)(p22;p24),? del(21)(q21q22),+2 mar	*JAK2:* RP11-927H16 *PCM1:* RP11-484L21	*PCM1:* exon 24; *JAK2:* exon 15	intensive CHT	No	ND	multiple vertebral tumors
10	Murati et al.	43	M	CEL	t(8;9)(p21;p24)	*JAK2:* RP11-927H16 *PCM1:* RP11-484L21	No	HU, INF, allo-BMT	ND	ND	
11	Murati et al.	30	M	MDS/MPN	t(8;9)(p22;p24),del(12)(p13p13)	*JAK2:* RP11-927H16 *PCM1:* RP11-484L21	*PCM1:* exon 23; *JAK2:* exon 10	HU, IFN, splene-ctomy	No	ND	
12	Heiss et al.	61	M	MDS/MPN	t(8;9)(p23;p24)	Yes, probes not specified	No	ND	ND	ND	prominent erythoid dysplasia/ hyperplasia; myelofibrosis, eosinophilia, progression to EL

Table 1. (Continued)

Case n.	Ref.	Age (y)	Gender	Diagnosis	Cytogenetics	FISH	RT-PCR	Therapy	Achievment of CyR	Achievment of MoIR	Peculiar features
13	Bousquet et al.	46	M	aCML	t(8;9) (p22;p24)	*JAK2:* RP11-927H16 *PCM1:* RP11-484L21	*PCM1:* exon 37; *JAK2:* exon 9	HU, allo-BMT	ND	ND	
14	Bousquet et al.	44	M	AML	t(8;9) (p22;p24)	*JAK2:* RP11-927H16 *PCM1:* RP11-484L21	No	intensive CHT	ND	ND	supra-clavicular mass, eosino-philia, likely evolution from aCML
15	Adélaïde et al.	40	M	T-cell lymph-oma	t(8;9) (p22;p24)	Yes, probes not specified	*PCM1:* exon 37; *JAK2:* exon 9	intensive CHT+ CNS radiotherapy, auto-BMT after relapse	Yes	Yes (assess-ed after inten-sive CHT)	
16	Huang et al.	48	F	AML	t(8;9) (p22;p24)	*JAK2:* RP11-23O2 and RP11-60G18 *PCM1:* RP11-343L2 and RP11-3K23	No	intensive CHT	No	No	translocation acquired during relapse associated with express-ion of HLA-DR

Case n.	Ref.	Age (y)	Gender	Diagnosis	Cytogenetics	FISH	RT-PCR	Therapy	Achievment of CyR	Achievment of MolR	Peculiar features
17	Dargent et al.	57	M	aCML	t(8;9) (p22;p24)	*JAK2:* RP11-125K10 and RP11-639K24	No	ND	ND	ND	erythroid dysplasia, eosinophilia, ↓MKpoiesis, reticulin +
18	Lierman et al.	72	M	CEL	t(8;9) (p22;p24)	*JAK2:* RP11-307I14, RP11-125K10 and RP11-509D8 *PCM1:* RP11-140C18 and RP11-635N21	*PCM1:* exon 36; *JAK2:* exon 9	HU, ruxolitinib	Yes (CCyR)	ND	eosinophilia
19	Patterer et al.	73	M	AML	t(8;9) (p22;p24)	*JAK2:* RP11-509D8	*PCM1:* exon 35; *JAK2:* exon 9	Supportive care	No	No	BM hypoplasia
20	Patterer et al.	75	F	AML	t(8;9) (p21;p24),+13	Yes, probes not specified	*PCM1:* exon 35; *JAK2:* exon 9	Supportive care	No	No	
21	Patterer et al.	72	M	MDS/MPN	t(8;9) (p22;p24),del(6) (q16q26),	*JAK2:* RP11-509D8	*PCM1:* exon 28; *JAK2:* exon 11	HU	No	No	myelofibrosis, eosinophilia
22	Patterer et al.	50	M	MPN	t(8;9) (p22;p24)	Yes, probes not specified	*PCM1:* exon 35; *JAK2:* exon 9	Ruxolitinib	ND	ND	eosinophilia

Table 1. (Continued)

Case n.	Ref.	Age (y)	Gender	Diagnosis	Cytogenetics	FISH	RT-PCR	Therapy	Achievment of CyR	Achievment of MoIR	Peculiar features
23	Patterer et al.	47	M	AML	der(1)t(1;8)(p36;q22), der(5)t(5;17)(q22;q21), t(8;9)(p22;p24),+ider(9)(p10)t(8;9)(p12;p24)	Yes, probes not specified	*PCM1*: exon 35; *JAK2*: exon 9. *PCM1*: exon 28; *JAK2*: exon 9	intensive CHT	No	No	eosinophilia
24	Patterer et al.	50	M	B-ALL	der(8)t(8;9)(p21;24) t(8;22)(q24;q21), der(9)t(8;9)(p21;24), der(21)t(1;21)(q21;p11), der(22)t(8;22)(q24;q11)	Yes, probes not specified	*PCM1*: exon 35; *JAK2*: exon 9	intensive CHT	CCyr only for t(8;22), persistence of t(8;9)	No	likely evolution of MPN, progressive disease

Case n.	Ref.	Age (y)	Gender	Diagnosis	Cytogenetics	FISH	RT-PCR	Therapy	Achievment of CyR	Achievment of MolR	Peculiar features
25	Rumi et al.	31	F	CEL-NOS	t(8;9) (p22;p24)	*JAK2:* RP11-3H3 and RP11-963L3 *PCM1:* RP11-880I6 and RP11-428L21	*PCM1:* exon 36; *JAK2:* exon 9	HU, ruxolitinib	Yes (from ~50% to ~30% of positive meta-phases) at 1 y	Yes (~75% reduc-tion)	eosinophilia, erythroid dysplasia, myelofibrosis
26	Masselli et al.	29	M	aCML	t(8;9) (p22;p24)	*JAK2:* RP11-125K10 and RP11-39K24 *PCM1:* RP11-156K13 and RP11-428L21	*PCM1:* exon 25; *JAK2:* exon 9	INF, intensive CHT, allo-BMT	Yes (only after allo-BMT)	Yes (only after allo-BMT)	erythroid dysplasia
27	Saba et al.	35	M	MPN	t(8 ;9) (p22 ;p24)	ND	No	ND	ND	ND	

One of the most intriguing aspect of this heterogeneous group of diseases is related to the peculiar abnormalities of the erythroid lineage that typifies a remarkable percentage of the reported cases (18.5%, see patient n. 9, 12, 17, 25 and 26) [30, 34-35, 37, 39]. This observation is even more relevant if we consider that the cytogenetic abnormality involves JAK2, which detains a pivotal role in signal transduction down-stream the EPO receptor. Histopathological features may range from erythroid dysplasia (cases n. 17, 25 and 26) [30, 34, 37] to overt erythroid leukemia (patients n. 9 and 12) [35, 39]. Erythroid dysplasia is characterized by large nodules of immature erythoid precursors (mainly proerythroblasts and early erythroblasts), with high mitotic activitiy and impaired differentiative capacity. They are typically localized in paratrabecular areas with a pronounced microvessel density. Since normal erythropoiesis is not physiologically found at the paratrabecular spaces, the unique distribution of these clusters of morphologically abnormal proerythroblasts can be interpreted, as observed by Heiss et al. [39], as a sign of dysplasia, similarly to what described for myelopoiesis in myelodysplastic syndromes (the so called "ALIP", Abnormal Localized Immature Precursors).

If the pathophysiological bases of this erythroid dysplasia might be related to the involvement of the JAK2-signaling is not clear yet.

Our group for first investigated the behavior, in-vitro, of CD34$^+$ hematopoietic progenitors from a t(8;9)(p22;p24)/*PCM1-JAK2* MDS/MPN presenting with aCML and prominent erythroid dysplasia (abundant large peritrabecular clusters of proerythroblasts associated with marked reduction of the mature erythroid compartment) (see case n.26). CD34$^+$ cells were cultured for 14 days in serum-free medium supplemented with recombinant human interleukin-3 (rIL-3), stem cell factor (SCF) and EPO to induce erythroid differentiation. Cell growth and erythroid output (assessed as percentage of Glycophorin A-positive cells by flow cytometric analysis) were compared to a healthy subject (HD) and a PV patient, bearing the constitutively-active *JAK2*V617F mutation that drives autonomous cell proliferation and erythroid differentiation.

We found that CD34$^+$ from the *PCM1-JAK2* fusion patient displayed impaired growth (F.I.= 0.6 vs 8 of PV and 6.5 of HD) and erythroid differentiation capacity, as demonstrated by the low percentage of Glycophorin A-positive cells (3.1% vs 84.5% of PV and 52.6% of HD), suggesting a phenotype distinct from *JAK2V617F*-positive PVs. Additionally, we proved that the *in-vitro* behavior of primary CD34$^+$ cells from our patient faithfully reproduce the *in-vivo* dyserythropoietic phenotype of the bone marrow [34].

Whether *PCM1-JAK2* fusion-associated malignancies arise in hematopoietic stem-cells compartment or in lineage-committed progenitors has not been determined yet. However, our experimental data, together with the lack of a clear lineage-specificity (both myeloid and lymphoid malignancies are described) are consistent with the idea that the PCM1-JAK2 disease, similarly to CML, originates from a hematopoietic stem cell.

Cytogenetic Aspects

Chromosome break points are identified by FISH as p22 on chromosome 8 and p24 on chromosome 9 in the vast majority of the patients (17 out of 27 cases, 63%), followed by p21 on chromosome 8 and p24 on chromosome 9 (6 out of 27 cases, 22%). Only two cases (8%) of break points located at p23 on chromosome 8 and p24 on chromosome 9 and at p22 on chromosome 8 and p23 on chromosome 9 have been described.

A complex karyotype, with the *PCM1-JAK2* translocation being part of multiple chromosomal abnormalities, is not uncommon (cases n. 6, 9, 11, 20, 23, 24) [19, 35-36]. No phenotype-specificity can be described, but similarly to other hematologic malignancies (AML and MDS in particular), a rapidly progressive clinical course is observed, such as death early after diagnosis (case n. 6) [19] or during induction chemotherapy (case n. 20) [36], early relapse (patient n. 23 and 24) [36] and association with other tumors (patient n. 9) [35].

Molecular Aspects

Biological properties of the chimeric PCM1-JAK2 protein are topic of ongoing studies. All the translocation variants with alternative break-points on the short arms of chromosome 8 and 9 that have been described so far (see previous paragraph) preserve the N-terminal domain of PCM1 and the C-terminal domain of JAK2.

The N-terminal domain of PCM1 is characterized by the presence of multiple coiled-coil motifs, while the C-terminus of JAK2 contains the kinase (JH1) and pseudokinase (JH2) domain. Bousquet et al. and Murati et al. hypothesized, in 2005, that this peculiar structure of the fusion protein facilitates oligomerization of the PCM1-JAK2 chimera resulting in a constitutive activation of JAK2 [29, 35]. However, if PCM1 multiple coiled-coil domains serve as dimerization motifs to induce JAK2 autophosphorylation has never been proved yet.

Lierman et al. demonstrated that, similarly to what described for *ETV6-JAK2* and *SEC31A-JAK2* fusions, BaF3 cells (a murine fibroblast cell line) expressing *PCM1-JAK2* display an activated JAK-STAT axis and that treatment with the JAK-inhibitor ruxolitinib leads to impaired cell growth and reduced phosphorylation of JAK2 and STAT5 [33].

Ehrentraut and colleagues investigated the signaling potentially down-stream PCM1-JAK2 fusion in a trio of human lymphoma cell lines (MAC-1/2A/2B) carrying the t(8;9), showing up-regulation of Suppressor Of Cytokine Signaling 2 and 3 (SOCS2 and 3, two negative regulators of JAK2 signaling) after *PCM1-JAK2* lentiviral knock-down and pharmacological inhibition by a JAK2-inhibitor (TG101348). Additionally, similarly to Lierman et al., they observed a robust phosphorylation of STAT3 and 5 but treatment with TG101348 was not able to reduce (as in the case of STAT3) or induced only a moderate reduction at very high doses (as in the case of STAT5) of STAT proteins [31].

Given this background, our group analyzed, in primary cells from a patient presenting with t(8;9)(p22;24)/*PCM1-JAK2* aCML, the activation pattern of the three main signaling cascades activated by JAK2: Mitogen-activated protein (MAP) kinase, JAK/STAT and PI3K/Akt pathway.

Circulating neoplastic cells harboring the fusion transcript were subjected to western blot analyses with antibodies that separately recognize the total and phosphorylated (i.e. activated) forms of JAK2, STAT3, STAT5, Akt and ERK1/2. We found reduced levels of phosphorylated STAT3, total and phosphorylated JAK2, STAT5 and Akt, and a robust increase in ERK1/2 phosphorylation. These results indicate that PCM1-JAK2 fusion protein is incapable of activating the JAK/STAT signaling axis but may selectively activate ERK1/2 pathway.

Intriguingly, this aspect was consistent not only with the clinical and histopathological features of this patient, indicative of a myeloproliferative stimulus associated with erythroid dysplasia, but also with in-vitro behavior of CD34$^+$ hematopoietic progenitors described above [34].

Our data provide the first evidence *in-vivo* that ERK1/2, rather than JAK/STAT axis, is the signaling pathway primarily activated in *PCM1-JAK2* fusion-related diseases with erythroid dysplasia and immediately pinpoint to a potential druggable target in the subset of patients resistant to JAK-inhibitors.

Clinical Course and Treatment

PCM1-JAK2-related hematologic malignancies present an aggressive clinical course and poor outcome. Four out of 27 patients (14,8%) died within one month since the time of diagnosis, because of rapidly progressive disease (see patient n. 3, 6 and 19) [19, 36] or during induction chemotherapy (patient n. 4 and 19) [19, 36]. Collectively, 9 patients died within 1 year since the time of diagnosis, mainly due to relapse/refractory disease.

Several therapeutic approaches have been adopted, ranging from a conservative treatment, based on supportive care or low dose cytoreductive therapy (i.e. hydroxyurea, interferon-α) for elderly patients, to more aggressive treatments including intensive chemotherapy and allogenic bone marrow transplant for "fit" patients. Based on the rationale that t(8;9) involves a TK, efficacy of Imatinib has been assessed in 2 cases (n. 8 and 25), described by Murati et al. [35] and Rumi et al. [37], respectively. Unfortunately, similarly to what described for *FGFR1* translocations, they had a very poor response, supporting the idea that only patients carrying rearrangements of *BCR-ABL*, *PDGFRA* and *PDGFB* respond to Gleevec®.

Intensive chemotherapy regimens are usually extremely toxic and poorly tolerated, with a very low percentage of long-term response (see cases n. 4, 16, 23 and 24) [19, 32, 36], and we believe they must be considered only in those patients eligible for transplant who require, consequently, disease de-bulking.

Allogenic bone marrow transplant (BMT) is the only curative options, but, unfortunately, only the minority of patients is candidate for this type of treatment because of age, comorbidities and HLA-matched suitable donors. BMT was performed in 6 out of 27 patients (22,2%, see cases n. 5, 7, 10, 13, 15 and 26) [19, 28-29, 34-35], of which 5 were allogenic BMT and only 1 autologous BMT (patient n. 15) [28]. Median age was 41 years (range 29-46 years). One patient died because of transplant-related mortality (case n. 13) [29] while the others were still alive and progression-free at the time of publication (83%). Concerning the patients who could not benefit from BMT, only 5 out of 19 (26%) were alive when data were assembled. Although numbers are low and no statistical consideration can be drawn, these observations suggest that early allogenic BMT should be considered for eligible *PCM1-JAK2*-positive patients with a suitable donor.

Very few data concerning treatment response are available, mainly because of the short follow-up and the rapid disease progression. Cytogenetic response was assessed in 18 patients, while molecular response was provided only in 9 cases. Only 4 cases were able to achieve a cytogenetic response. Surprisingly, one of these patients was treated with the sole interferon-α (case n. 2) [19]. Our study is the first providing a complete cytogenetic and molecular monitoring after BMT. In our case, the sole chemotherapy wasn't able to reduce the number of metaphases carrying the t(8;9) and, consistently, nested RT-PCR documented persistence of the fusion transcript both in bone marrow and peripheral blood mononuclear cells. Only the allogenic BMT was able to restore a normal karyotype and to clear the pathological transcript [34].

Data on molecular response are scant. Only 3 patients experienced a reduction/clearance of the PCM1-JAK2 fusion transcript (patients n. 15, 25 and 26) [28, 34, 37]. In case n. 15, the presence of chimeric transcript was assessed by RT-PCR after induction chemotherapy in peripheral blood and bone marrow mononuclear cells, revealing a complete clearance [28]. Rumi et al. monitored fusion transcript by quantitative real-time PCR from granulocytes after 3, 6 and 12 months of treatment with ruxolitinib, reporting a reduction at approximately 20% of the baseline value [37]. We evaluated the molecular response of our patients by nested RT-PCR from peripheral blood and bone marrow mononuclear cells after the first and second course of chemotherapy and at +100 days after allo-BMT, showing a complete clearance of the *PCM1-JAK2* fusion gene only after transplantation [34].

A new, promising therapeutic approach is offered by the recent approval of the JAK1/2 inhibitor ruxolitinib for "classic" Philadelphia-negative MPN and, specifically, for high risk myelofibrosis. The fact that the PCM1-JAK2 chimeric protein retains the TK domain of JAK2 provided a molecular target for the treatment with this oral JAK-inhibitor. Although very few experiences have been reported so far (3 patients in total), preliminary data suggest that ruxolitinib is an effective drug, capable to induce cytogenetic responses (a complete cytogenetic response for patient n. 18 and a partial cytogenetic response for patient n. 25) [33, 37]. No information about therapy response are available for patient n. 22 [36]. Interestingly, a similar response was obtained also in one case treated with interferon-α, as described by Reiter et al. [19]. Only Rumi and colleagues provided an evaluation of the molecular response under ruxolitinib, with a ~75% of reduction of the *PCM1-JAK2* fusion transcript [37].

CONCLUSION

PCM1-JAK2-related hematologic malignancies are rare disorders, characterized by a broad clinical spectrum, a rapid evolution and a dismal prognosis. Current therapeutic options are limited and allogenic bone marrow transplant remains the only curative treatment for eligible patients.

Great hopes have been raised since the introduction of the oral JAK-inhibitor ruxolitinib, which has been used in the last two years in three cases with achievement of cytogenetic responses (one CCyR and one PCyR)[33, 37]. However, longer follow-up as well as larger data sets from clinical trials are eagerly awaited. Unfortunately, the scientific community has to deal with small numbers and heterogeneous diseases.

More efforts need to be done also on the "bench side", to elucidate the mechanisms of activation of PCM1-JAK2 fusion protein and to pinpoint the down-stream events that lead to neoplastic transformation. Hopefully, future studies will help identifying new molecular targets to address with "tailored" therapeutic approaches.

ABBREVIATIONS

aCML	atypical chronic myeloid leukemia
AL	acute leukemia
ALL	acute lymphoblastic leukemia
Allo-BMT	allogenic bone marrow transplant
AML	acute myeloid leukemia
Auto-BMT	autologous bone marrow transplant
CEL	chronic eosinophilic leukemia
CEL-NOS	chronic eosinophilic leukemia-not otherwise specified
CHT	chemotherapy
CNS	central nervous system
CyR	cytogenetic response
CCyr	complete cytogenetic response
EL	erythroid leukemia
HU	hydroxyurea
INF	interferon
MKpoiesis	megakaryocytopoiesis
MDS	myelodysplastic syndromes

MPN	myeloproliferative neoplasm
MolR	molecular response
ND	not determined
PCyR	partial cytogenetic response

REFERENCES

[1] Nowell, PC; Hungerford, DA. Chromosome studies on normal and leukemic human leukocytes. *J Natl Cancer Inst*, 1960 Jul, 25, 85-109.

[2] Rowley, JD. Letter: A new consistent chromosomal abnormality in chronic myelogenous leukaemia identified by quinacrine fluorescence and Giemsa staining. *Nature*, 1973 Jun 1, 243(5405), 290-3.

[3] Tefferi, A; Vardiman, JW. Classification and diagnosis of myeloproliferative neoplasms: the 2008 World Health Organization criteria and point-of-care diagnostic algorithms. *Leukemia*, 2008 Jan, 22(1), 14-22.

[4] Walz, C; Cross, NC; Van, Etten, RA; Reiter, A. Comparison of mutated ABL1 and JAK2 as oncogenes and drug targets in myeloproliferative disorders. *Leukemia*, 2008 Jul, 22(7), 1320-34.

[5] Peeters, P; Raynaud, SD; Cools, J; Wlodarska, I; Grosgeorge, J; Philip, P; et al. Fusion of TEL, the ETS-variant gene 6 (ETV6), to the receptor-associated kinase JAK2 as a result of t(9;12) in a lymphoid and t(9;15;12) in a myeloid leukemia. *Blood*, 1997 Oct 1, 90(7), 2535-40.

[6] Lacronique, V; Boureux, A; Valle, VD; Poirel, H; Quang, CT; Mauchauffe, M; et al. A TEL-JAK2 fusion protein with constitutive kinase activity in human leukemia. *Science*, 1997 Nov 14, 278(5341), 1309-12.

[7] Griesinger, F; Hennig, H; Hillmer, F; Podleschny, M; Steffens, R; Pies, A; et al. A BCR-JAK2 fusion gene as the result of a t(9;22) (p24;q11.2) translocation in a patient with a clinically typical chronic myeloid leukemia. *Genes Chromosomes Cancer*, 2005 Nov, 44(3), 329-33.

[8] Hoeller, S; Walz, C; Reiter, A; Dirnhofer, S; Tzankov, A. PCM1-JAK2-fusion: a potential treatment target in myelodysplastic-myeloproliferative and other hemato-lymphoid neoplasms. *Expert Opin Ther Targets*, 2011 Jan, 15(1), 53-62.

[9] Nebral, K; Denk, D; Attarbaschi, A; Konig, M; Mann, G; Haas, OA; et al. Incidence and diversity of PAX5 fusion genes in childhood acute lymphoblastic leukemia. *Leukemia*, 2009 Jan, 23(1), 134-43.

[10] Poitras, JL; Dal, Cin, P; Aster, JC; Deangelo, DJ; Morton, CC. Novel SSBP2-JAK2 fusion gene resulting from a t(5;9)(q14.1;p24.1) in pre-B acute lymphocytic leukemia. Genes Chromosomes *Cancer*, 2008 Oct, 47(10), 884-9.

[11] Dammermann, A; Merdes, A. Assembly of centrosomal proteins and microtubule organization depends on PCM-1. *J Cell Biol*, 2002 Oct 28, 159(2), 255-66.

[12] Brinkley, BR. Microtubule organizing centers. *Annu Rev Cell Biol*, 1985, 1, 145-72.

[13] Rose, MD; Biggins, S; Satterwhite, LL. Unravelling the tangled web at the microtubule-organizing center. *Curr Opin Cell Biol*, 1993 Feb, 5(1), 105-15.

[14] Kalt, A; Schliwa, M. Molecular components of the centrosome. *Trends Cell Biol*, 1993 Apr, 3(4), 118-28.

[15] Kubo, A; Sasaki, H; Yuba-Kubo, A; Tsukita, S; Shiina, N. Centriolar satellites: molecular characterization, ATP-dependent movement toward centrioles and possible involvement in ciliogenesis. *J Cell Biol*, 1999 Nov 29, 147(5), 969-80.

[16] Balczon, R; Bao, L; Zimmer, WE. PCM-1, A 228-kD centrosome autoantigen with a distinct cell cycle distribution. *J Cell Biol*, 1994 Mar, 124(5), 783-93.

[17] Hames, RS; Crookes, RE; Straatman, KR; Merdes, A; Hayes, MJ; Faragher, AJ; et al. Dynamic recruitment of Nek2 kinase to the centrosome involves microtubules, PCM-1, and localized proteasomal degradation. *Mol Biol Cell*, 2005 Apr, 16(4), 1711-24.

[18] Balczon, R; Simerly, C; Takahashi, D; Schatten, G. Arrest of cell cycle progression during first interphase in murine zygotes microinjected with anti-PCM-1 antibodies. *Cell Motil Cytoskeleton*, 2002 Jul, 52(3), 183-92.

[19] Reiter, A; Walz, C; Watmore, A; Schoch, C; Blau, I; Schlegelberger, B; et al. The t(8;9)(p22;p24) is a recurrent abnormality in chronic and acute leukemia that fuses PCM1 to JAK2. *Cancer Res*, 2005 Apr 1, 65(7), 2662-7.

[20] Vizmanos, JL; Novo, FJ; Roman, JP; Baxter, EJ; Lahortiga, I; Larrayoz, MJ; et al. NIN, a gene encoding a CEP110-like centrosomal protein, is fused to PDGFRB in a patient with a t(5;14)(q33;q24) and an imatinib-responsive myeloproliferative disorder. *Cancer Res*, 2004 Apr 15, 64(8), 2673-6.

[21] Corvi, R; Berger, N; Balczon, R; Romeo, G. RET/PCM-1: a novel fusion gene in papillary thyroid carcinoma. *Oncogene*, 2000 Aug 31, 19(37), 4236-42.

[22] Quintas-Cardama, A; Kantarjian, H; Cortes, J; Verstovsek, S. Janus kinase inhibitors for the treatment of myeloproliferative neoplasias and beyond. *Nat Rev Drug Discov*, 2011 Feb, 10(2), 127-40.

[23] Shi, S; Calhoun, HC; Xia, F; Li, J; Le, L; Li, WX. JAK signaling globally counteracts heterochromatic gene silencing. *Nat Genet*, 2006 Sep, 38(9), 1071-6.

[24] Levine, RL; Wadleigh, M; Cools, J; Ebert, BL; Wernig, G; Huntly, BJ; et al. Activating mutation in the tyrosine kinase JAK2 in polycythemia vera, essential thrombocythemia, and myeloid metaplasia with myelofibrosis. *Cancer Cell*, 2005 Apr, 7(4), 387-97.

[25] Kralovics, R; Passamonti, F; Buser, AS; Teo, SS; Tiedt, R; Passweg, JR; et al. A gain-of-function mutation of JAK2 in myeloproliferative disorders. *N Engl J Med*, 2005 Apr 28, 352(17), 1779-90.

[26] James, C; Ugo, V; Le, Couedic, JP; Staerk, J; Delhommeau, F; Lacout, C; et al. A unique clonal JAK2 mutation leading to constitutive signalling causes polycythaemia vera. *Nature*, 2005 Apr 28, 434(7037), 1144-8.

[27] Scott, LM; Tong, W; Levine, RL; Scott, MA; Beer, PA; Stratton, MR; et al. JAK2 exon 12 mutations in polycythemia vera and idiopathic erythrocytosis. *N Engl J Med*, 2007 Feb 1, 356(5), 459-68.

[28] Adelaide, J; Perot, C; Gelsi-Boyer, V; Pautas, C; Murati, A; Copie-Bergman, C; et al. A t(8;9) translocation with PCM1-JAK2 fusion in a patient with T-cell lymphoma. *Leukemia*, 2006 Mar, 20(3), 536-7.

[29] Bousquet, M; Quelen, C; De, Mas, V; Duchayne, E; Roquefeuil, B; Delsol, G; et al. The t(8;9)(p22;p24) translocation in atypical chronic myeloid leukaemia yields a new PCM1-JAK2 fusion gene. *Oncogene*, 2005 Nov 3, 24(48), 7248-52.

[30] Dargent, JL; Mathieux, V; Vidrequin, S; Deghorain, X; Vannuffel, P; Rack, K. Pathology of the bone marrow and spleen in a case of myelodysplastic/myeloproliferative neoplasm associated with t(8;9)(p22;p24) involving PCM1 and JAK2 genes. *Eur J Haematol*, 2011 Jan, 86(1), 87-90.

[31] Ehrentraut, S; Nagel, S; Scherr, ME; Schneider, B; Quentmeier, H; Geffers, R; et al. t(8;9)(p22;p24)/PCM1-JAK2 activates SOCS2 and SOCS3 via STAT5. *PLoS One*, 2013, 8(1), e53767.

[32] Huang, KP; Chase, AJ; Cross, NC; Reiter, A; Li, TY; Wang, TF; et al. Evolutional change of karyotype with t(8;9)(p22;p24) and HLA-DR immunophenotype in relapsed acute myeloid leukemia. *Int J Hematol*, 2008 Sep, 88(2), 197-201.

[33] Lierman, E; Selleslag, D; Smits, S; Billiet, J; Vandenberghe P. Ruxolitinib inhibits transforming JAK2 fusion proteins in vitro and induces complete cytogenetic remission in t(8;9)(p22;p24)/PCM1-JAK2-positive chronic eosinophilic leukemia. *Blood*, 2012 Aug 16, 120(7), 1529-31.

[34] Masselli, E; Mecucci, C; Gobbi, G; Carubbi, C; Pierini, V; Sammarelli, G; et al. Implication of MAPK1/MAPK3 signalling pathway in t(8;9)(p22;24)/PCM1-JAK2 myelodysplastic/ myeloproliferative neoplasms. *Br J Haematol*, 2013 Aug, 162(4), 563-6.

[35] Murati, A; Gelsi-Boyer, V; Adelaide, J; Perot, C; Talmant, P; Giraudier, S; et al. PCM1-JAK2 fusion in myeloproliferative disorders and acute erythroid leukemia with t(8;9) translocation. *Leukemia*, 2005 Sep, 19(9), 1692-6.

[36] Patterer, V; Schnittger, S; Kern, W; Haferlach, T; Haferlach, C. Hematologic malignancies with PCM1-JAK2 gene fusion share characteristics with myeloid and lymphoid neoplasms with eosinophilia and abnormalities of PDGFRA, PDGFRB, and FGFR1. *Ann Hematol*, 2013 Jun, 92(6), 759-69.

[37] Rumi, E; Milosevic, JD; Casetti, I; Dambruoso, I; Pietra, D; Boveri, E; et al. Efficacy of ruxolitinib in chronic eosinophilic leukemia associated with a PCM1-JAK2 fusion gene. *J Clin Oncol*, 2013 Jun 10, 31(17), e269-71.

[38] Saba, N; Safah, H. A myeloproliferative neoplasm with translocation t(8;9)(p22;p24) involving JAK2 gene. *Blood*, 2013 Aug 8, 122(6), 861.

[39] Heiss, S; Erdel, M; Gunsilius, E; Nachbaur, D; Tzankov, A. Myelodysplastic/myeloproliferative disease with erythropoietic hyperplasia (erythroid preleukemia) and the unique translocation (8;9) (p23;p24): first description of a case. *Hum Pathol*, 2005 Oct, 36(10), 1148-51.

In: Myeloproliferative Disorders
Editor: Anthony M. Camden

ISBN: 978-1-63321-201-5
© 2014 Nova Science Publishers, Inc.

Chapter 4

SYMPTOMS, RISK FACTORS AND TREATMENT OPTIONS OF MYELOPROLIFERATIVE NEOPLASMS

Fabiola Attié de Castro[1,*], *Ph.D., Hematology Professor,*
Sandra Mara Burin[1,**],
Daniela Dover de Araujo[1,2,†], *Ph.D.,*
Natalia de Souza Nunes[1,‡],
Mariana Cristina Lima Souza[3,§],
Cristiane Fernandes de Freitas Tavares[1,4,#], *Ph.D., and*
Raquel Tognon Ribeiro[5,††], *Ph.D., Hematology Professor*

[1]Clinical Analyses, Toxicology and Food Sciences Department, School of Pharmaceutical Science of Ribeirão Preto-University of São Paulo, Ribeirão Preto, Brazil
[2]University of Educational Foundation of Guaxupé - UNIFEG, Minas Gerais, Brazil

---

[*] Email: castrofa@fcfrp.usp.br.
[**] Email: sandra_burin@yahoo.com.br.
[†] Email: danydover@hotmail.com.
[‡] Email: natisnunes@gmail.com.
[§] Email: mariana_lima88@hotmail.com.
[#] Email: cfftavares@hotmail.com.br.
[††] Email: raqueltognon.ribeiro@ufjf.edu.br.

[3]Department of Hematology,
Federal University of São Paulo/ São Paulo, Brazil
[4]University of Franca, UNIFRAN, Franca, São Paulo, Brazil
[5]Department of Pharmacy, Federal University of Juiz de Fora/Governador
Valadares Campus, Governador Valadares, Brazil

ABSTRACT

The myeloproliferative neoplasms (MPN) are hematological diseases characterized by a myelo accumulation and clonal myeloproliferation of mature myeloid cells, which means peripheral blood granulocytosis, erythrocytosis and thrombocytosis.

The World Health Organization (WHO), in 2008, revised the criteria for classification and diagnosis of chronic myeloid neoplasms and now the Myeloproliferative Neoplasms (MPN) category includes chronic myelogenous leukemia (CML), polycythemia vera (PV), essential thrombocythemia (ET), primary myelofibrosis (PMF), chronic neutrophilic leukemia (CNL), chronic eosinophilic leukemia not otherwise categorized, hypereosinophilic syndrome (HES), mast cell disease (MCD) and MPN unclassified. This chapter will focus on diagnosis criteria, symptoms, risk factors and treatment options of myeloproliferative neoplasms, specifically CML, PV, and PMF.

The CML diagnosis is based on blood counts (leukocytosis and frequently also thrombocytosis) and the presence of circulating immature granulocytes, from the metamyelocyte to the myeloblast, and basophilia. Splenomegaly may be detected in >50% of patients in the initial chronic phase (CP), but 50% of patients are asymptomatic. Diagnosis is finally obtained by the observation of the Philadelphia (Ph) chromosome (22q-) and/or the *BCR-ABL1* oncogene in peripheral blood or bone marrow cells. CML is a tryphasic disease and the prognostic scores (Sokal and Hasford) were calculated based on patiens´age, spleen size and blood cell counts. Other patient characteristics must be considered in CML risk groups with a different prognosis, such as a different response rate, a different progression-free survival and a different overall survival, also for patients treated with imatinib. CML treatments currently used are hydroxyurea, tyrosine-quinase inhibitors (imatinib, dasatinib and nilotinib) and bone marrow transplantation. The WHO diagnostic criteria for the classic *BCR-ABL*-negative diseases, PV, ET and PMF, were based on cell myeloproliferation, morphologic and cytochemical features in bone marrow (biopsy and myelogram) as well as molecular findings (JAK2 and MPL mutations). In addition, other criteria are required for distinguishing the MPN subtypes for patients negative for JAK2 mutation. PV and ET patients present a high risk of thrombosis and a late risk of clonal evolution into PMF or acute myeloid leukemia (AML). PMF patients may also present a high risk of progressing to AML. The relations among laboratorial or molecular data and clinical features have been extensively studied and, as a consequence, the risk stratification, the risk-adapted therapy definition and systems for prognosis prediction have been improved for MPN patients. Besides the description of relative efficacy of many unspecific drugs for MPN, the molecular mechanisms discovery has made the development of target therapy with tyrosine kinases inhibitors possible. Many of them are in the final phase of clinical studies and some are already in clinical use.

1. BACKGROUND

The myeloproliferative neoplasms (MPN) are hematological diseases characterized by a myelo accumulation and clonal myeloproliferation of mature myeloid cells, which means peripheral blood granulocytosis, erythrocytosis and thrombocytosis.

The term "Chronic Myeloproliferative Diseases" (cMPD) was used the first time by William Dameshek in 1951, being defined at that time as hematological diseases with similar phenotypic characteristics, preserved cell hyperproliferation and maturation of one or more myeloid cells. In this group of diseases were grouped chronic myeloid leukemia (CML), polycythemia vera (PV), essential thrombocythemia (ET), primary myelofibrosis (PMF) and eritroleukemia [1, 2]. In 2001, the World Health Organization (WHO) cMPD classification included the disease classified by Dameshek and also hypereosinophilic syndrome / chronic eosinophilic leukemia (HES/CEL), the chronic neutrophilic leukemia (CNL) and Chronic MPD unclassifiable (3).

In 2008, the nomenclature of this group was changed for Myeloproliferative Neoplasms (MPN) and it was included under the systemic mastocytosis disease group. The WHO 2008 uses the cell morphology, cytochemistry analysis, the cell immunophenotype, genetics and patients clinical features as criteria for cMPD classification [4, 5]. The inclusion of molecular parameters in diagnosis criteria increase the sensitivity and specificity of the diagnosis of these pathologies to help in clinical practice but bone marrow biopsies still provide very useful information about marrow cellularity, topography, stromal changes, and maturation pattern of the hematopoietic lineages, being very important for disease follow-up during and after treatment. As highlighted by Vardiman (2008), it is important to emphasize that for WHO, the term "myeloid" includes all cells belonging to the granulocytic (neutrophil, eosinophil, basophil), monocytic/macrophage, erythroid, megakaryocytic and mast cell lineages, and that the WHO criteria for myeloid neoplasms applies to initial diagnostic peripheral blood (PB) and bone marrow (BM) specimens obtained prior to any definitive therapy for a suspected hematologic neoplasm [5].

The Chronic Myeloid Leukemia (CML) is a MPN characterized by the presence of the Philadelphia chromosome (Ph), which is the result of a reciprocal chromosomal translocation between the *C-ABL* (Abelson leukemia virus) oncogene on chromosome 9 and the *BCR* (breakpoint cluster region) on chromosome 22. The Ph chromosome encodes a *BCR-ABL1* neogene, which encodes a Bcr-Abl oncoprotein with a constant tyrosine kinase (TK) activity [6]. Among MPN, only CML is characterized by having an oncogene resulting from the fusion of the BCR and ABL genes (Ph chromosome positive) while PV, ET and PMF are known as Ph or BCR-ABL negatives diseases. Regarding PV, ET and PMF, the discovery of the mutation in the tyrosine kinase, Janus kinase 2 (JAK2) in 2005, has expanded the knowledge of the pathogenesis of Ph negative NPM, which allowed a better understanding of the molecular basis of NPM [7-9].

This chapter will focus on diagnosis criteria, symptoms, risk factors and treatment options of myeloproliferative neoplasms, specifically CML, PV, ET and PMF.

2. CHRONIC MYELOID LEUKEMIA

Among the leukemia that affects adults, CML is responsible for approximately 20% of cases in the West with an incidence of 1-2 cases per 100,000 inhabitants per year. It is more common in men than women and the incidence increases with age. In most cases it occurs after age 50 [10, 11]. The one major risk factor is the exposure to ionizing radiation and that is why it was observed that Japanese survivors of the atomic bomb had significantly increased risks [12, 13]. A slight increase of this risk was also observed in some patients undergoing high dose of radiotherapy for the treatment of other cancers, such as lymphoma [14, 15].

The CML diagnosis depends on the stage of the disease, but most of the patients are diagnosed at the chronic phase. At the chronic phase the patient diagnosis is initially made by a peripheral blood exam, which must show leukocytosis with granulocyte left shift, normal or elevated platelets counting, and symptoms indicative of spleen and/or liver enlargement. Some patients (<10%) may be diagnosed during the accelerated or blastic phases with bleeding, petechiae and ecchymosis and infections. The CML diagnosis confirmation is performed by the cytogenetic analysis of blood cells or bone marrow, where the Philadelphia chromosome (Ph) can be found in approximately 90% of the cases [16]. The fluorescent in situ hybridization (FISH) technique is more sensitive than classical cytogenetic, and makes it possible to analyze hundreds of cells through specific probes directed at the translocated gene [17]. The molecular biology techniques, such as real time Polymerase chain reaction (PCR) is used to detect and quantify the *BCR-ABL1* gene [18].

The absence of the Philadelphia chromosome and the *BCR – ABL1* gene excludes the diagnosis of CML.

Early CML diagnosis is performed by a blood exam analysis, presenting leukocytosis and thrombocytosis. In 80% of CML cases the related signs and symptoms are fever, weight loss, anorexia, weakness, and anemia and are associated with persistent abdominal pain, the rest of the cases are asymptomatic. At advanced CML stages, the patients may present blasts in the peripheral blood, and the increase of basophils and eosinophils [19].

The World Health Organization (WHO) has established a criteria for the CML three phases: chronic, accelerated and phase blast [20, 5]. Most of the patients´ diagnoses are made in the chronic stable phase, half of the patients are asymptomatic, and when symptoms are presented, they are generally related to hypercatabolism (weight loss, fatigue, fever and night sweats) and splenomegaly (feeling of satiety). In most cases the patients at this stage lives around 3-5 years. In 5% of cases the blood clotting may be abnormal, with excessive bleeding in minor injuries or during surgical procedures. The chronic phase (CP) can be divided into early and late phases [21]. In the positive "initial chronic phase" the BCR-ABL clones are expanding within the bone marrow and differentiate into mature cells [22, 23]. At this stage, some lymphoid and myeloid cells circulating hold the *BCR- ABL1* oncogene. In CP, it is very frequent to detect mutations in the ABL portion of the SH1 domain as well as in DNA breaks derived from cytogenetic abnormalities acquired with or without treatment, but still with clinical manifestations in the chronic phase [21].

The accelerated phase (AP) may occur months or years after diagnosis of the disease, depending on the response of the patient to the treatment in CP. The signs of deterioration are: fever, fatigue, weight loss, appearance of bone pain and a significant increase in the spleen, the presence of 1% to 19% blasts in blood or bone marrow being necessary, basophils number of >20%, and thrombocytosis or thrombocytopenia unrelated to therapy. This transition marks cytogenetic abnormalities in leukemic clones that respond to treatment, particularly due to mutations in the ATP binding site SH1 domain of *BCR-ABL* [23].

The blast crisis (BC) is characterized by increased blasts (> 20%) in bone marrow and peripheral blood leukocytosis, anemia and thrombocytopenia [24, 25]. The patient shows clinical signs of evolving such as being more susceptible to infection, anemia aggravation and the appearance of signs of hemorrhage. At this stage, the failure occurs in the maturation of malignant myeloid or lymphoid precursors, which often has cytogenetic alterations leading to CML aggravation [26, 27]. Although it is known that the effect of BCR-ABL is related to disease transformation, cellular and molecular mechanisms responsible for the onset and progression of CML that lead into AP/BC have not been completely elucidated yet [26].

The prognosis of CML is directly related to the phase of the disease at diagnosis, the method used for disease diagnosis and the treatment applied (or interferon-alpha inhibitors on first and second generation of TK), as well as the deletion associated with ABL and the type of mosaicism that occurs with the Ph chromosome. The type of deletion of ABL interferes in the survival. However, the worse prognosis is linked to Ph chromosome mosaicism [28]. The TK inhibitors lead to better results in the early phase of the disease and according the progression of the disease to AP or BC, and the overall and disease-free survival decrease [29, 30].

Sokal and Hasford created similar score predictions for CML. These scores are used nowadays in order to identify in CML patients on CP phase the risk for disease progression. They are calculated according the disease clinical and laboratory characteristics and the results, are expressed as: low, intermediate and high risk to disease progression. The Sokal score analyzes the spleen size in cm, the number of platelets, the percentage of blasts and age, where the result < 0.8 corresponds to 39% of CML patients at low risk, 0.8 to 1.2 corresponds to intermediate risk in 38% of patients, and > 1.2 corresponds to high risk in 23% of patients. This score has been widely used in patients with CML treated with imatinib, where the cytogenetic and molecular responses are higher in low-risk patients [31].

The Hasford score was developed for patients treated with alpha-interferon and analyzes the patients´ age, the percentage of eosinophils, basophils, platelet count, spleen size in centimeters and percentage of blasts. The Hasford scores are expressed as low risk when the result is ≤ 780 (40 % of patients), intermediate risk between 780 and 1480 (45 % of patients) and high risk ≥ 1480 (15% of patients) [32].

The CML treatment was performed by chemotherapeutic agents as busulfan and hydroxyurea. These agents were used for many years and helped to avoid the expansion of the myeloid tissue, providing clinical maintenance and improving the quality of life during the CP of the disease, but failed to eliminate the malignant clone in advanced phases such as AP and BC [33, 34]. In the mid-1970s, the introduction of allogeneic stem cell transplantation (alloSCT) marked the first important advance in the evolution and the outcome of CML, because the disappearance of the Ph-positive clone was reported in patients submitted to alloSCT and they were cured [25, 35]. Unfortunately, the alloSCT was successful in patients under 40 years old, whereas the median age of patients diagnosed was near 60 years, and the cure was commonly associated to development of a chronic graft-versus-host-disease (cGVHD) [36, 37, 33]. In the early 1980s, the introduction of interferon-alpha (INF-α) was considered another advance to clinical treatment, which led to complete cytogenetic response and long-term survival, but not in all patients [38, 39].

After conventional therapies, the increase knowledge of the abnormal activity of the BCR-ABL protein and its role in CML led to the development of molecules that targeted and inhibited the TK activity [40, 41].

The CML therapy was revolutionized in 2001, with the discovery of the tyrosine kinase inhibitor (TKI) imatinib mesylate (IM) (Gleevec, Novartis), becoming the first-line of CML therapy [42]. IM showed a high effectiveness in patients with CML at CP, inducing over 95% of complete hematological response and 73% of complete cytogenetic remission [43]. Although IM therapy is effective, IM-resistant cell clones have been described in patients treated in advanced phases. Furthermore, only about 65% of the patients with CML in advanced phases display hematological responses, and actually, it is known that there are also cases of IM resistance in patients at the chronic phase (21, 44, 45). Soon after IM, the second-generation of TK inhibitors (TKIs) such as Dasatinib (Sprycel, Bristol-Myers Squibb), Nilotinib (Tasigna, Novartis), Bosutinib (Busulif, Pfizer), and third-generation as Ponatinib (Iclusig, Ariad), were developed and tested and now used for CML patients with intolerance and/or resistance to IM [33, 46, 47]. Dasatinib and nilotinib have been demonstrated to be effective, with the possibility of reaching about 50% of patients with different kinds of resistance. Bosutinib effectiveness was also demonstrated in patients resistant to therapy with IM, dasatinib and/or nilotinib. All of these drugs are not effective in patients with CML positive for T315I mutations. Ponatinib was tested with interesting results, and it was lately approved for patients with resistance to other TKIs. This compound proved to be effective for the majority of patients with T315I mutation, as maintained by most of the responses [46, 48, 49]. Unfortunately, these compounds are not all available worldwide and the elevated prices are a problem that can hinder their use [47, 48]. In 2013, the European Leukemia Net (ELN) group published recommendations, in which alloSCT should be considered a possibility at the time of starting the second line and after unsuccess of any type of TKIs. However, it is recommended for patients after failure of two previous TKIs [49].

An appropriate cytogenetic and molecular monitoring can help in choosing the proper TKI and to optimize therapy. The inadequate intervention in the diagnosis and clinical treatment of CML with TKIs can lead to disease progression. Even in the mighty TKIs era, the survival after the progression into AP/BC is still too low [50-52].

3. PHILADELPHIA-NEGATIVE MPN

As described above, Polycythemia Vera (PV), Essential Thrombocythemia (ET) and Primary Myelofibrosis (PMF) are known as Ph (chromosome) or BCR-ABL negatives MPN. Until 2008, when WHO provided the last diagnosis criteria for MPN, the most commonly recognized mutation in BCR-ABL1–negative MPN was JAK2 V617F. The description of this mutation in 2005 led to an expansion in Ph negative NPM pathogenesis knowledge and allowed a better understanding of the molecular basis of NPM [53, 54].

The JAK family of protein kinases consists of four members (JAK1, JAK2, JAK3 and TYK2) that bind to cytokine receptors in the cytosolic domain. JAK2 has an important role in the signaling pathway for cytokine receptors on myeloid cells by binding to homodimeric type 1 receptors for erythropoietin, thrombopoietin, granulocyte colony stimulating factor [55]. The JAK kinases own two highly homologous domains in the carboxy terminal piece: a domain with kinase activity (JH1, JAK homology) and another pseudokinase inactive domain (JH2), the latter being a negative regulator of kinase activity JH1 [56].

The JAK2V617F mutation is specific and characterized by the exchange of guanine for thymine at nucleotide 1849 of exon 14 of the gene (chromosome 9), and the amino acid substitution of valine for phenylalanine occurring at position 617. The exchange of amino acids occurs in the area of pseudokinase JH2, resulting in loss of control of the self-inhibitory kinase domain of the JH1 over JH2 domain, leading to constitutive activation of the protein and thus hyperproliferation of erythrocytes, granulocytes and precursor thrombocytes [55, 56]. The JAK2 V617F mutation was found in 95% of patients with PV and in 50% of patients with ET and PMF. A small percentage of patients JAK2 V617F negative can have exon 12 mutations in the JAK2 gene with similar function in the JH2 field [57]. Additional molecular events may interfere with the JAK2 kinase activity, as deletion of chromosome 20 (20q-) and trisomy of chromosome 9 [56].

Later, in 2006, another molecular abnormality found in NPM is a somatic mutation at codon 515 of the MPL. The MPL is the receptor of cytokine thrombopoietin (TPO) expressed in hematopoietic precursors and cells of the megakaryocytic lineage. The two most frequent mutations are W515L, when substitution of amino acid tryptophan to leucine occurs, and the W515K mutation where the amino acid tryptophan is substituted by lysine, reported in 5 to 10% of patients with the PMF and W515L mutation and approximately W515K in 9% of patients with ET and in patients without the JAK2 mutation V617F14 [58]. The evolution of molecular knowledge of the JAK2 mutation reflects the progress of new therapeutic drugs in an attempt to block the progression of the disease.

The next topics will describe the diagnosis, symptoms, risk factors, prognosis and treatment options for PV, ET and PMF.

3.1. Polycythemia Vera

Polycythemia Vera is a MPN characterized by clonal proliferation of myeloid cells with predominance of red cells. According to WHO 2008 criteria for PV classification, major and minor criteria should be evaluated and the diagnosis will be PV when both major criteria and one minor or the first major criteria and two minor were filled. The major criteria includes: hemoglobin 18.5 g/dL in men and 16.5 g/dL in women or other evidence of increased red cell volume and presence of JAK2V617F mutation or similar mutation like JAK2 exon 12. Minor criteria include: bone marrow biopsy showing hypercellularity (panmyelosis) with prominent erythroid proliferation, serum erythropoietin (EPO) level below the reference, and endogenous erythroid colony formation in vitro [59].

Around 96% of PV patients harbor the JAK2V617F mutation and a higher allele burden was associated with pruritus and fibrotic transformation.

Normally patients are diagnosed at an older age with a higher hemoglobin level, leukocytosis and a lower platelet account harbor JAK2V617F mutation while, the exon 12 mutation is representative of younger people and lower serum erythropoietin level. Initially it was believed that PV prognosis was similar in both conditions with or without JAK2V617 mutation [59]. However, recent studies show that the allele burden could be an influence in disease development and can be used as patient monitoring. Alshemmari et al. showed that high allele burden levels are associated to patients with higher WBC and hemoglobin levels and low allele burden levels associated to high platelet levels [60].

Among the PV patients showing vascular disturbances, headache, splenomegaly and hepatomegaly, pruritus, erythromelalgia, hemorrhagic complications and/or fatigue, around 30% develop PMF and 10% progress towards for leukemic transformation. It has been shown that no differences were observed in thromboembolic events between JAK2V617 homozygous and heterozygous [61].

PV risk stratification is not associated with life expectancy, survival, leukemic/fibrotic transformation, or risk of complications. This stratification regards therapeutic treatment. Age > 60 years and history of thrombosis represents high risk, none of these factors are low risk, one of both represents intermediate risk [61, 62].

3.2. Primary Myelofibrosis

Primary Myelofibrosis (PMF) is a Philadelphia-negative clonal hematopoietic stem cell disorder characterized by intense reactive changes of bone marrow (BM) stroma with collagen fibrosis, osteosclerosis and angiogenesis [63].

The PMF is associated with the presence of JAK2V617F mutation in 50 to 60% of cases and MPL W515L/K mutation in less than 10% [58, 64]. Commonly, PMF affects elderly people, with an average age at diagnosis around 65 years old and less than 20% of the patients are younger than 50 years [65]. The clinical course of PMF varies from 1 to 30 years and may evolve from asymptomatic into progressive BM failure, symptomatic splenomegaly and risk of acute leukemia in 10-20% of cases [66, 67]. Actually, one third of PMF patients are asymptomatic at diagnosis and the remaining present progressive anemia, extramedullary hematopoiesis and constitutional symptoms such as loss of weight, fatigue and night sweats [68].

Table 1. PMF Risks and criteria of evaluation for each classification.

Classification	Criteria	Risks	References
DUPRIEZ (Lille)	Hemoglobin < 10 g/dL WBC <4 or >30x10^9/L	0= Lo 1= Intermediate 2 = High	Dupriez et al, 1996 [71]
CERVANTES	Hemoglobin < 10 g/dL Constitutional Symptoms* Circulating Blasts > 1%	0 -1 = Low 2- 3 = High	Cervantes et al, 1998 [72]
MAYO	Hemoglobin < 10 g/dL Platelets < 100 x10^9/L WBC <4 or > 30 x10^9/L Mono > 1 x10^9/L	0= Low 1= Intermediate >2= High	Tefferi et al, 2007 [73]
IPSS (Internacional Prognostic Scoring System)	Age > 65 years Hemoglobin < 10 g/dL WBC > 25 x10^9/L Circulating Blasts >/= 1% Constitutional Symptoms*	0= Low 1= Intermediate-1 2=Intermediate-2 >3=High	Cervantes et al, 2009 [65]
DIPSS-PLUS (Dynamic International Prognostic Scoring System- Plus)	Age > 65 years Hemoglobin < 10 g/dL WBC > 25 x10^9/L Circulating Blasts >/= 1% Constitutional Symptoms* Unfavorable Karyotype** Platelets < 100 x10^9/L Red Cell Transfusion	0=Low 1=Intermediate-1 2-3=Intermediate-2 >4= High	Gangat et al, 2011 [75]

WBC: white blood counts, mono: monocytes; * Constitutional symptoms included nights sweats, fever, weight loss.

** Unfavorable Karyotype included complex karyotype or single or two abnormalities, including +8,-7/7q-, i(17q),-5/5q-, 12p-, inv(3) or 11q23 rearrangement.

Source: Adapted from Souza, MC et al. Application of five prognostic survival scores to Primary Myelofibrosis in 62 Brazilian patients. Medical Oncology, 2013; April (30:555). [104].

Patients with PMF have normochromic, normocytic anemia and mild reticulocytosis. Typically, the patients present at peripheral blood smear the tear-drop shape blood cells, elliptocytes, poikilocytosis, and erythrocytic and granulocytic precursors in peripheral blood. The myelogram is usually hypocellular or dry, with a possible increase in the number of megakaryocytes [4].

In PMF, the fibrosis is due to clonal proliferation of hematopoietic cells that leads to hyperplasia of megakaryocytes and monocytes that release fibrogenic growth factor [69].

The treatment plan is designed individually for each person, according to his or her characteristics and disease. The main goal of therapy is to prolong survival since cure can be achieved only by a minority of patients who are candidates for allogeneic hematopoietic stem cell transplant (HSCT) [71]. As new drugs and diverse transplant options have been developed it is useful to identify patients with different life expectancies in order to select those that may benefit from each therapeutic alternative. PMF risk stratification is based on parameters predicting survival and several attempts have been made to identify clinical and laboratory features that could predict patients' survival. Among the available prognostic scores for risk stratification are: Lille [71], Cervantes [72], Mayo [73], IPSS [65], DIPSS [74] and DIPSS-Plus [75] (Table 1).

In the nineties, Dupriez et al (1996) studied the survival of 195 PM patients and detected hemoglobin <10g/dL and white blood cell (WBC) count <4 or >30×10^9/L were able to distinguish patients in three groups (low, intermediate and high risks), associated with a median survival of 93, 26 and 13 months, for each group [71]. Dupriez´s scoring system, also named Lille, was simple and useful for survival estimation. However, for young patients there was no specific prognostic data. In order to gain a better understanding of the disease in younger patients, Cervantes et al, (1998) conducted a collaborative study with 550 patients <55 years old, and identified three variables independently associated with shorter survival: Hb<10g/dL; presence of constitutional symptoms (fever, sweats, weight loss) and circulating blasts >1% [72]. Two groups were identified: low risk, in which PM had an indolent course (median survival of 176 months) and high risk (median survival 33 months). This scoring system has a high positive predictive value for the young group. More recently, Tefferi et al, (2007) at Mayo Clinic, added two more prognostic factors to the Lille score: monocytosis > 1×10^9/L and thrombocytopenia (platelets <100×10^9/L) and found a better hazard ratio profile that could identify higher life expectancy patients as well as delineate the intermediate risk category [76]. However, even with the contributions of these systems, they failed to adequately separate intermediate and poor prognosis patients.

The International Prognostic Scoring System (IPSS) was then created by the International Working Group for Myelofibrosis Research and Treatment, studying 109 patients diagnosed from 1980, with a median age of 63 years, and classified according to WHO criteria [77, 78, 79]. The features independently associated with poor prognosis were age >65years, constitutional symptoms, hemoglobin (Hb) <10g/dL, WBC count > $25x10^9$/L and >1% blasts in peripheral blood. IPSS presented a higher discriminating power than previous scoring systems as well as replicability and accuracy [66]. However, as the IPSS was recorded at diagnosis a system that could reflect the variations occurring during disease progression was necessary. In this way, a score called DIPPS could be applied any time in the course of the disease, because it may be able to predict the patient's life expectancy and to guide the physicians to the best therapy to be adopted [74]. To develop DIPSS, 525 patients were studied and the same risk factors were recorded with diverse weighting, upgrading the scores [79, 80]. DIPSS was updated when three new parameters were inserted, changing its name to DIPSS-Plus. The parameters were: thrombocytopenia $<100x10^9$/L, need for red blood cell transfusion and unfavorable karyotype (i.e. complex, or one of the abnormalities: +8-7/7q-,i(17q),-5/5q-,12p-,inv(3), or 11q23 rearrangement).

3.3. Essential Thrombocythemia

Essential Thrombocythemia (ET) is a MPN characterized by an excessive proliferation of megakaryocytes with marked increase of platelet numbers [81]. In 2008, WHO established the diagnosis criteria for ET, which included clinical, morphological and molecular characteristics [4]. An ET diagnosis requires the presence of the 4 major criteria: (1) Platelets count higher than 450 x 10(9)/L; (2) Megakaryocyte proliferation with large and mature morphology and no or little granulocyte or erythroid proliferation; (3) not meeting WHO criteria for CML, PV, PMF, MDS or other myeloid neoplasm; (4) demonstration of JAK2V617F or other clonal marker or no evidence of reactive thrombocytosis [4, 5].

Considering morphological criteria, patients presenting ET may be separated into two groups: the first is called 'true ET' and the second early/prefibrotic PMF. This has been a challenge for the clinicians, since the distinction is based on clinically distinctive and specific histological BM patterns and the reproducibility and clinical usefulness of this classification of chronic myeloproliferative neoplasm (MPN) persist to be a controversial issue [82].

The differential diagnosis with PMF or secondary thrombocytosis is very important for the diagnosis. Some findings are essential in this subject but some of them are still a challenge in clinical practice. Recent works have shown that it is not frequent to find a relevant increased bone marrow cellularity or a significant increase in proliferation or a left-shifting of the neutrophil granulo- or erythropoiesis in true ET whereas randomly distributed clustered of megakaryocytes with hyperlobulated nuclei can be frequently visualized, leading to doubts. However, a very helpful characteristic in ET is that a very small number of patients have an accumulation of reticulin fibers in the bone marrow whereas in early prefibrotic PMF, histopathology of the bone marrow is characterized by hematopoietic hypercellularity consisting of a prominent neutrophil granulocytic and megakaryocytic proliferation, which is often associated with a slight to moderate reduction of nucleated red cell precursors. Additionally, in PMF is usually visualized in an abnormal arrangement and localization in the marrow and a high variability in size is found as well as significant aberrations of nuclear organization [82]. Molecular-genetic findings as JAK2V617F mutation may help to exclude reactive thrombocytosis, although in ET and PMF only 50-60% of the cases show JAK2 V617F. Other studies have been investigating other mutations for proposing molecular markers, such as MPL, TET2 and ASXL1, but they are not exclusive of ET. A new mutation in the CALR gene was recently identified in JAK2 V617F and MPL W515 negative ET patients and could be included in the future as molecular markers [83, 84]. Many authors have been raising a discussion about the difficulties in differential diagnosis. A study performed by Buhr et al (2012), which enrolled 102 cases of ET and PMF, compared clinical criteria with histopatological evaluation independently performed by six hematopathologists [85]. This group concluded that criteria for discrimination of ET from prefibrotic PMF are poorly to only moderately reproducible and led to a higher proportion of non-classifiable myeloproliferative neoplasms than histology alone [88]. However, Barbui et al (2013) argue that other recently published retrospective and prospective clinical pathologic studies featuring the WHO criteria provided important information on disease outcomes, supporting the existence of early/prefibrotic PMF as a distinct clinical pathologic entity in patients presenting clinically with ET. For example, Koopmans et al. reported that a significantly high degree of consensus (83%) was obtained for the WHO-defined individual major histological features, particularly megakaryocytes, in their study with MPN patients. Corroborating this opinion, Wilkins et al. (2008) found an agreement on the final histological classification of about 70% [86]. Barbui et al (2013) believes that studies on MPN without adequate clinical and morphological input with no compliance with the concept of the WHO classification leads to controversies and suggested that it is necessary to a scientific project, including the community of pathologists and hematologists, in order to provide sound, objective and reproducible criteria for diagnosing early/prefibrotic PMF [82].

Other studies are still looking for markers to differentiate ET and secondary thrombocytosis. Mignon et al (2013) performed a study about the expression of molecules involved in the coagulation process and found that patients with reactive thrombocytosis had a longer lag time, higher endogenous thrombin potential, peak of thrombin generation and velocity index than patients with essential thrombocythemia [87]. They also found that the level of circulating procoagulant phospholipids was increased in patients with ET. For differentiating JAK2-mutated ET from masked PV more easily, some hematological parameters have been proposed as feasible markers. Barbui et al (2014) found in a recent work that hemoglobin and hematocrit thresholds of masked PV patients were significantly higher than JAK2V617F ET and suggested that the best cut-off for hemoglobin to discriminate JAK2-mutated ET from PV was 16.5 g/dL for males and 16.0 g/dL for females [88]. Regarding hematocrit, the cut-off was 49% in males and 48% in females, reaching a proportion of correct diagnosis with these parameters of 95% in males and 93% in females [88].

The ET incidence is about 2,5/100.000/ year and it is more prevalent in woman than man [89]. Many ET patients do not present significant symptoms, but others can show symptoms as erythromelalgia, hemorrhage, transient ischemic attacks (including reversible ischemic neurologic defects), microvascular ischemia of the digits, as well as a variety of constitutional symptoms, including headache, visual disturbances, chronic fatigue, and pruritus [83]. In 2007, a survey of 1,179 MPN patients was published and showed that these patients do indeed suffer from excessive fatigue compared to age-matched controls and that symptoms compromise social functioning, physical activity, independence in daily tasks, and global quality of life [90]. Another study of the same group evaluated 17 independent symptoms present among an MPN population and found that the prevalence and severity of symptoms varied widely between MPN subtypes (range in prevalence 17% -

59% for ET, 18% - 68% for PV, and 29% - 77% for MF), suggesting that heterogenetic phenotypes exist [91].

Survival of ET patients does not substantially differ from that of the general population. However, important morbidity is derived from vascular complications, including thrombosis, microvascular disturbances, and bleeding [92]. The ET patients that can be classified as high risk match the following criteria: age higher than 60 years, previous history of thrombosis and high risk of bleeding if platelet counts are >1500 x 10(9)/L. A prognostic model to predict survival named IPSET (International Prognostic Score for ET) developed by Passamonti et al (2012) studying 867 ET patients according to WHO diagnosis criteria. Considering factors as age >60y, leukocytes count > 11 x 10(9)/L and history of thrombosis, the patients were allocated into 3 risk categories with significantly differential survival: low (no adverse points), intermediate (1 or 2 adverse points) and high (3 or more adverse points) risk categories, with corresponding median survivals of 'not reached', 25 years and 14 years. This system was further validated in independent cohorts including 132 ET patients, confirming that this model is able to predict the occurrence of thrombosis but not to predict myelofibrosis transformation [93]. The International Working Group for MPN Research and Treatment (IWG-MRT) studies have also identified platelet count of 1.000x10(9)/L and thrombosis history as predictors of leukemic transformation, and absence of JAK2V617F, older age and anemia as predictors of progression into overt PMF [94].

Other risk factors have been investigated. According to Campbell et al (2012), no association was seen between blood counts at diagnosis and future complication in a longitudinal study with 21,887 individuals. However, this group found associations between platelet counts outside of the normal range during follow-up and immediate risk of major hemorrhage but not thrombosis and elevated WBC count during follow-up was correlated with thrombosis [95]. Chou (2013) found that splenomegaly in essential thrombocythemia is an independent risk factor for hemorrhage [96]. Montanaro et al (2014) identified independent prognostic factors for shorter thrombosis-free survival: age higher than 60 years, previous thrombosis and at least one cardiovascular risk. For overall survival, this group found age higher than 60 years, anemia, male gender, previous thrombosis and white blood cell count higher than 15 x 10(9)/L [97]. The JAK2 V617F has also been proposed as a risk factor for vascular events and myelofibrotic transformation in polycythemia vera and essential thrombocythemia. For further investigation, Alvarez-Larran et al (2014) performed a JAK2 V617F monitoring during follow-up of 347 PV and ET patients in order to correlate the evolutionary patterns and vascular events

[98]. According to this group, the multivariate analyses, patients with a persistently higher or unsteady JAK2 V617F allele burden had an increased risk of myelofibrotic transformation and a trend for a higher incidence of thrombosis than patients with a stable allele burden below 50% [98]. The impact of the calreticulin (CARL) mutation, described recently, over the clinical and hematological phenotype and outcome in ET patients has been studied. Rotunno (2013) found that patients carrying CALR mutation had a lower risk of thrombosis than JAK2 and MPL mutated ET. This author also verified that CARL mutation seems to have no impact on survival or myelofibrosis transformation and conclude thatmore studies are still necessary in this field [84].

3.4. PV, ET and PMF Treatment

The treatment for PV, ET and PMF patients depends on the risk classification of the patient and therefore it must be designed individually for each person, according to their characteristics and disease. The main goal of therapy is therefore to prevent thrombohemorrhagic events and control systemic symptoms.

The therapy for PV patients included in low/intermediate-risk stratification is usually phlebotomies. This procedure serves to reduce the RBC mass and blood viscosity, improve platelet function, increase plasma volume, restore systemic and pulmonary pressures, and decrease the risk of thrombotic events [83]. Low dose aspirin is frequently used in these cases also, for alleviating thrombotic disturbances. High-risk PV patients' stratification should be treated with cytoreductive therapy, with Hydroxyurea (HU) or IFN-α as the first line choice [99]. HU is also the first choice for high-risk ET patients. However, it has been described that PV and ET patients are developing resistance or intolerance to HU [98, 100]. In this case, busulfan, interferon-α, pipobroman and anagrelide are possible choices for second-line therapy [60, 100]. For PMF, as mentioned above, cure can be achieved only by a minority of patients who are candidates for allogeneic hematopoietic stem cell transplant (HSCT) [70]. If the patient is not a suitable HSCT candidate, the treatment plan may include observation only; drug therapies, removal of the spleen; radiotherapy or possible participation in clinical studies [70]. All treatment options should be discussed between the patient and the medical staff. In the case of relevant comorbidities or higher age (>65 years), erythropoiesis-stimulating agents may be used for anemia control in PMF

[102]. Androgens (danazol), immunomodulators (thalidomide/lenalidomide), splenectomy, splenic irradiation, INF, and cytoreductive therapy (such as HU, busulfan, and melphalan) have been also used in patients with PMF to address leukocytosis or thrombocytosis, marked splenomegaly, and constitutional symptoms [83].

Regarding thrombohemorrhagic events in PV and ET, whether a general cytoreductive (ie, leukocyte-reducing) effect, rather than a selective platelet-lowering effect discussion is still ongoing. Some studies observed that the platelet-lowering effect of HU is associated with a lower rate of thrombotic complications, suggesting that high-risk patients should receive cytoreductive therapy with hydroxyurea and that platelet counts could serve as a surrogate marker for clinical complications [103]. A retrospective investigation observed that an increased leukocyte count at diagnosis of ET was associated with thrombosis during follow-up and therefore, the leukocyte-lowering effect of hydroxyurea could reduce thrombosis [103].

Anagrelide, a recommended second-line treatment option for patients with high-risk ET, blocks megakaryocyte differentiation and proliferation and inhibits cyclic AMP phosphodiesterase activity. In combination with aspirin, it was associated with increased rates of arterial thrombosis, serious hemorrhage and transformation to PMF. Additionally, higher rates of side effects decrease the treatment adherence. However, this drug also has advantages, for example treated patients showed a significantly lower incidence of venous thromboembolism [99]. A prospective randomized single-blind phase 3 study performed by Gisslinger et al (2013) compared the efficacy, tolerability, and safety of anagrelide and hydroxyurea in a homogeneous cohort of patients with ET diagnosed according to the WHO classification. They did not find any significant difference between the anagrelide and hydroxyurea group regarding thrombosis, bleeding or rates of discontinuation. They also did not observe disease transformation into myelofibrosis or secondary leukemia in this study. The results indicate that anagrelide, as a selective platelet-lowering agent, is not inferior compared with hydroxyurea in the prevention of thrombotic complications in ET patients [103]. Gugliota et al (2013) investigated a cohort of 3,643 patients, and described 9.5% of these patients had received combined therapy: 87.6% of them receiving hydroxycarbamide + anagrelide and before this combination, 54.9% of the patients had received monotherapy with hydroxycarbamide and 40.5% with anagrelide. According to this study, median weekly doses of hydroxycarbamide and anagrelide were 7000 and 10.5 mg when used as prior monotherapy and 3500 and 7.0 mg when used as add-on treatment and a reduction in platelet count was observed by using the combination [101].

Pipobroman, busulfan and radioactive phosphorus are also recommended as second-line agents for patients after failure of primary therapy with either HU or IFN-α. However, due to the potential leukemogenicity of these agents, these agents should be reserved for patients with more than 80 years [101]. A pegylated form of IFN- α shows antiproliferative effects on hematopoietic precursor cells, inducing cytogenetic remissions and reducing the JAK2 V617F allele burden in MPNs though it shows intolerable side effects, including flulike symptoms, fatigue and neuropsychiatric symptoms, leading to high rates of discontinuation. More recently, newer PEGylated formulations of IFN- α (PEG-IFN), which are better tolerated and allow for less frequent administration, have renewed interest in IFN- α as a therapeutic option for patients with PV and ET [99].

After the JAK2 V617F mutation description in 2005, the search for JAK2 inhibitors started. The developed inhibitors have demonstrated remarkable activity in patients with PMF and post-PV/ post-ET MF. The first JAK inhibitor approved by the US Food and Drug Administration (FDA) was Ruxolitinib® to treat PMF and nowadays has being studied in patients with PV and ET who are refractory to or intolerant of HU, with a starting dose of 10 mg (for PV) or 25 mg (for ET) twice daily, with dose adjustments allowed as necessary. New agents for myeloproliferative neoplasms have been studied. For example, histone deacetylase (HDAC) inhibitors are being tested in patients with PV and ET that are resistant to HU. The combination HDAC inhibitor Givanostat with HU was well tolerated. The authors suggest that a strategy combining lower, potentially less toxic doses of HDAC inhibitors with other therapies, such as HU or JAK inhibitors, could be tested in patients with treatment-refractory PV or ET [99].

To evaluate treatment response, the criteria established by the European Leukemia Network (ELN) in 2009 seems not to predict clinically relevant endpoints. This association has now revised the response criteria for PV and ET, defining Complete Response (CR) as white blood cell count (WBC) <10x10(9) /L, platelet count <400 x10(9) /L normal spleen size on imaging and absence of disease-related symptoms; for PV, hematocrit < 45% without phlebotomy is an additional criterion. In addition, specific evaluation of symptomatic improvement and histological bone marrow changes were included, along with the required durability of response and four response categories were defined. For evaluation of CR: (1) resolution of disease signs and improvement in symptoms for at least 12 weeks; (2) normalization of peripheral blood for at least 12 weeks; (3) absence of vascular events and disease progression; and (4) disappearance of bone marrow histological abnormalities. For partial response (PR), the first three criteria are considered, but do not require the remission of bone-marrow histological abnormalities. Although some therapies have been shown to reduce the JAK2 *V617F* allele burden, molecular remission was not included in the revised response definition, given, for example, that nearly half of patients with ET lack the JAK2 V617F mutation, and remission of the JAK2 V617F clone has not been definitely shown to correlate with eradication of the disease [99, 100].

REFERENCES

[1]   Dameshek W. Some speculations on the myeloproliferative syndromes. *Blood.* 1951;6(4):372-5.

[2]   Tefferi A, Thiele J, Vardiman JW. The 2008 World Health Organization classification system for myeloproliferative neoplasms: order out of chaos. *Cancer.* 2009;115(17):3842-7.

[3]   Vardiman JW, Harris NL, Brunning RD. The World Health Organization (WHO) classification of the myeloid neoplasms. *Blood.* 2002;100(7):2292-302.

[4]   Swerdlow SH, Campo, E., Harris, N. L., Jaffe, E. S., Pileri, S. A., Stein, H., Thiele, J., Vardiman, J.W. WHO Classification of Tumours of Haematopoietic and Lymphoid Tissue. Lyon, France: World Health Organization; 2008. 439 p.

[5]   Vardiman JW, Thiele J, Arber DA, Brunning RD, Borowitz MJ, Porwit A, et al. The 2008 revision of the World Health Organization (WHO) classification of myeloid neoplasms and acute leukemia: rationale and important changes. *Blood.* 2009;114(5):937-51.

[6]   Deininger MW, Vieira S, Mendiola R, Schultheis B, Goldman JM, Melo JV. BCR-ABL tyrosine kinase activity regulates the expression of multiple genes implicated in the pathogenesis of chronic myeloid leukemia. *Cancer Res.* 2000;60(7):2049-55.

[7]   Milosevic JD, Kralovics R. Genetic and epigenetic alterations of myeloproliferative disorders. *Int. J. Hematol.* 2013;97(2):183-97.

[8]   Delhommeau F, Pisani DF, James C, Casadevall N, Constantinescu S, Vainchenker W. Oncogenic mechanisms in myeloproliferative disorders. *Cell Mol. Life Sci.* 2006;63(24):2939-53.

[9]   Levine RL, Wadleigh M, Cools J, Ebert BL, Wernig G, Huntly BJ, et al. Activating mutation in the tyrosine kinase JAK2 in polycythemia vera, essential thrombocythemia, and myeloid metaplasia with myelofibrosis. *Cancer Cell.* 2005;7(4):387-97.

[10]   Rohrbacher M, Hasford J. Epidemiology of chronic myeloid leukaemia (CML). *Best Pract. Res. Clin. Haematol.* 2009;22(3):295-302.

[11]   Cortez D, Kadlec L, Pendergast AM. Structural and signaling requirements for BCR-ABL-mediated transformation and inhibition of apoptosis. *Mol. Cell Biol.* 1995;15(10):5531-41.

[12]   Johnson KJ, Blair CM, Fink JM, Cerhan JR, Roesler MA, Hirsch BA, et al. Medical conditions and risk of adult myeloid leukemia. *Cancer Causes Control.* 2012;23(7):1083-9.

[13]   Tsushima H, Iwanaga M, Miyazaki Y. Late effect of atomic bomb radiation on myeloid disorders: leukemia and myelodysplastic syndromes. *Int. J. Hematol.* 2012;95(3):232-8.

[14]   Preston DL, Kusumi S, Tomonaga M, Izumi S, Ron E, Kuramoto A, et al. Cancer incidence in atomic bomb survivors. Part III. Leukemia, lymphoma and multiple myeloma, 1950-1987. *Radiat. Res.* 1994;137(2 Suppl):S68-97.

[15]   Bauduer F, Ducout L, Dastugue N, Marolleau JP. Chronic myeloid leukemia as a secondary neoplasm after anti-cancer radiotherapy: a report of three cases and a brief review of the literature. *Leuk. Lymphoma.* 2002; 43(5):1057–1060.

[16]   Zitzelsberger H[1], Bauchinger M, Wilmanns W, Strauss PGCytogenetic and molecular analysis of a "masked" Philadelphia chromosome in chronic and blastic phases of chronic myeloid leukemia. *Cancer Genet. Cytogenet.* 1990 Jul 15;47(2):219-25.

[17]   Landstrom AP[1], Tefferi A. Fluorescent in situ hybridization in the diagnosis, prognosis, and treatment monitoring of chronic myeloid leukemia. *Leukemia & Lymphoma.* 2006 Mar;47(3):397-402.

[18]   Tashfeen S, Ahmed S, Bhatti FA, Ali N. Real time polymerase chain reaction in diagnosis of chronic myeloid leukemia. *J. Coll. Physicians Surg. Pak.* 2014 Mar;24(3):190-3.

[19]   Jorge Cortes, MD. Natural history and staging of chronic myelogenous leukemia. *Hematol. Oncol. Clin. N. Am.* 2004; 18: 569–584.

[20]   Ahmed R, Naqi N, Hussain I, Khattak BK, Nadeem M, Iqbal J. Presentating phases of chronic myeloid leukaemia. *J. Coll. Physicians Surg. Pak.* 2009;19:469-72.

[21] Radich JP. Chronic myeloid leukaemia: where are we now and where can we go? *Hematology Am. Soc. Hematol. Educ. Program.* 2010;122-8.

[22] Melo JV, Barnes DJ. Chronic myeloid leukaemia as a model of disease evolution in human cancer. *Nat. Rev. Cancer.* 2007;7(6):441-53.

[23] Perrotti D, Jamieson C, Goldman J, Skorski T. Chronic myeloid leukemia: mechanisms of blastic transformation. *J. Clin. Invest.* 2010;120(7):2254-64.

[24] Faderl S, Kantarjian HM, Talpaz M. Chronic myelogenous leukemia: update on biology and treatment. *Oncology* (Williston Park). 1999;13(2):169-80.

[25] Hehlmann R, Hochhaus A, Baccarani M, LeukemiaNet E. Chronic myeloid leukaemia. *Lancet.* 2007;370(9584):342-50.

[26] Heaney NB, Holyoake TL. Therapeutic targets in chronic myeloid leukaemia. *Hematol. Oncol.* 2007;25(2):66-75.

[27] Cotta CV, Bueso-Ramos CE. New insights into the pathobiology and treatment of chronic myelogenous leukemia. *Ann. Diagn. Pathol.* 2007;11(1):68-78.

[28] Marzocchi G, Castagnetti F, Luatti S, Baldazzi C, Stacchini M, Gugliotta G, et al. Variant Philadelphia translocations: molecular-cytogenetic characterization and prognostic influence on frontline imatinib therapy, a GIMEMA Working Party on CML analysis. *Blood.* 2011;117:6793-800.

[29] Druker BJ, Guilhot F, O'Brien SG, Gathmann I, Kantarjian H, Gattermann N, et al. Five-year follow-up of patients receiving imatinib for chronic myeloid leukemia. *N. Engl. J. Med.* 2006;355(23):2408-17.

[30] Baccarani M, Dreyling M; ESMO Guidelines Working Group. Chronic myelogenous leukemia: ESMO clinical recommendations for diagnosis, treatment and follow-up. *Ann. Oncol.* 2009;20 (Suppl 4):105-7.

[31] Sokal JE, Cox EB, Baccarani M, Tura S, Gomez GA, Robertson JE et al. Prognostic discrimination in "good-risk" chronic granulocytic leukemia. *Blood.* 1984; 63: 789-99.

[32] Hasford J, Pfirrmann M, Hehlmann R, Allan NC, Baccarani M, Kluin-Nelemans JC et al. A new prognostic score for survival of patients with chronic myeloid leukemia treated with interferon alfa. *J. Natl. Cancer Inst.* 1998; 90: 850-8.

[33] Baccarani M, Castagnetti F, Gugliotta G, Palandri F, Rosti G. Treatment Recommendations for Chronic Myeloid Leukemia. *Mediterr. J. Hematol. Infect. Dis.* 2014 Jan 2;6(1): e2014005.

[34] Kantarjian HM, Larson RA, Cortés JE, Deering KL, Mauro MJ. Current practices in the management of chronic myeloid leukemia. *Clin. Lymphoma Myeloma Leuk.* 2013;13(1):48-54.

[35] Tohami T, Nagler A, Amariglio N. Laboratory tools for diagnosis and monitoring response in patients with chronic myeloid leukemia *Isr. Med. Assoc. J.* 2012 Aug;14(8):501-7.

[36] Agrawal M, Garg RJ, Kantarjian H, Cortes J. Chronic myeloid leukemia in the tyrosine kinase inhibitor era: what is the "best" therapy? *Curr. Oncol. Rep.* 2010; 12: 302-13

[37] Pavlu J, Szydlo RM, Goldman JM, and Apperley JF. Three decades of transplantation for chronic myeloid leukemia: what have we learned? *Blood.* Jan 20;117(3):755-63.

[38] Kantarjian HM, Smith TL, O'Brien S, Beran M, Pierce S, Talpaz M. Prolonged survival in chronic myelogenous leukemia after cytogenetic response to interferon-alpha therapy. The leukemia service. *Ann. Intern. Med.* 1995; 122: 254.

[39] Talpaz M, Hehlmann R, Quintas-Cardama A, et al. Re-emergence of interferon-α in the treatment of chronic myeloid leukemia. *Leukemia.* 2013 Apr;27(4):803-12.

[40] O'Brien SG, Guilhot F, Larson R, et al. Imatinib compared with interferon and low-dose cytarabine for newly diagnosed chronic-phase chronic myeloid leukemia. *N. Engl. J. Med.* 2003; 348:994-1004.

[41] Ferdinand R, Mitchell SA, Batson S, Tumur I. Treatments for chronic myeloid leukemia: a qualitative systematic review. *J. Blood Med.* 2012;3:51-76.

[42] Thienelt CD, Green K, Bowles DW. New and established tyrosine kinase inhibitors for chronic myeloid leukemia. *Drugs Today* (Barc) 2012;48:601–13.

[43] Weisberg E, Griffin J. Resistance to imatinib (Glivec): update on clinical mechanisms. *Drug Resist. Updat.* 2003;6:231–8.

[44] Gorre ME, Mohammed M, Ellwood K, Hsu N, Paquette R, Rao PN et al. Clinical resistance to STI571 cancer therapy caused by BCRABL gene mutation or amplification. *Science.* 2001;293:876 80.

[45] Azam M, Latek RR, Daley GQ. Mechanisms of auto inhibition and STI-571/imatinib resistance revealed by mutagenesis of BCR-ABL. *Cell* 2003;112:831–43.

[46] Saglio G, Kim DW, Issaragrisil S, et al. Nilotinib versus imatinib for newly diagnosed chronic myeloid leukemia. *N. Engl. J. Med.* 2010;362: 2251-9.

[47] Cortes JE, Kim DW, Pinilla-Ibarz J, et al. A phase 2 trial of ponatinib in Philadelphia chromosome-positive leukemias. *N. Engl. J. Med.* 2013; 369(19):1783-96.

[48] Cortes JE, Kantarjian H, Shah NP, et al. Ponatinib in refractory chromosome-positive leukemias. *N. Engl. J. Med.* 2012;367:2075-2088.

[49] Breccia M, Alimena G. Second-Generation Tyrosine Kinase Inhibitors (Tki) as Salvage Therapy for Resistant or intolerant Patients to Prior TKIs. *Mediterr. J. Hematol. Infect. Dis.* 2014; 6(1):e2014003.

[50] Baccarani M, Deininger MW, Rosti G, et al. European LeukemiaNet recommendations for the management of chronic myeloid leukemia: 2013. *Blood* 2013;122:872-84.

[51] Hehlmann R. How I treat CML blast crisis. *Blood* 2012;120:737-47.

[52] Haznedaroglu IC. Monitoring the Response to Tyrosine Kinase Inhibitor (TKI) Treatment in Chronic Myeloid Leukemia (CML). *Mediterr. J. Hematol. Infect. Dis.* 2014 Jan 1;6(1):e2014009.

[53] Delhommeau F, Pisani DF, James C, Casadevall N, Constantinescu S, Vainchenker W. Oncogenic mechanisms in myeloproliferative disorders. *Cell Mol. Life Sci.* 2006;63(24):2939-53.

[54] Cross NC. Genetic and epigenetic complexity in myeloproliferative neoplasms. *Hematology Am. Soc. Hematol. Educ. Program.* 2011;2011: 208-14.

[55] Yin CC. Medeiros LJ, Bueso-Ramos CE. Recent advances in the diagnosis and classification of myeloid neoplasms – comments on the 2008 WHO classification. *Int. Jnl. Lab. Hem*, v.32, p.461-476, 2010.

[56] Vainchenker W, Delhommeau F, Constantinescu SN, Bernard OA. New mutations and pathogenesis of myeloproliferative neoplasms. *Blood*, v.118, n.7, p.1723-1735, 2011.

[57] Jekarl DW, Han SB, Kim M, et al. JAK2 V617F mutation in myelodysplastic syndrome, myelodysplastic syndrome/ myeloproliferative neoplasm, unclassifiable, refractory anemia with ring sideroblasts with thrombocytosis and acute myeloid leukemia. *Korean J. Hematol.*, v.45, n.1, p.46-50, 2010.

[58] Pikman Y, Lee BH, Mercher T, et al. MPLW515L is a novel somatic activating mutation in myelofibrosis with myeloid metaplasia. *PLoS Med.* 2006; 3: 270.

[59] Silver RT, Chow W, Orazi A, Arles SP, Goldsmith SJ. Evaluation of WHO criteria for diagnosis of polycythemia vera: a prospective analysis. *Blood.* 2013 Sep 12;122(11):1881-6.

[60] Alshemmari SH, Rajaan R, Ameen R, Al-Drees MA, Almosailleakh MR. JAK2V617F allele burden in patients with myeloproliferative neoplasms. *Ann. Hematol.* 2013 Dec; 22.

[61] Tefferi A. Polycythemia vera and essential thrombocythemia: 2012 update on diagnosis, risk stratification, and management. *Am. J. Hematol.* 2012 Mar;87(3):285-93.

[62] Koopmans SM, van Marion AM, Schouten HC, et al. Myeloproliferative neoplasia: a review *Neth. J. Med.* 2012 May;70(4):159-67.

[63] Chauffaille ML. Alterações cromossômicas em síndrome mielodisplásica. *Rev. Bras. Hematol. Hemoter.* 2006;28(3):182-7.

[64] Pardanani AD, Levine RL, Lasho T, et al. MPL515 mutations in myeloproliferative and other myeloid disorders: a study of 1182 patients. *Blood.* 2006;108 (10):3472-6.

[65] Cervantes F, Dupriez B, Pereira A, et al. New prognostic scoring system for primary myelofibrosis based on a study of the International Working Group for Myelofibrosis Research and Treatment. *Blood.* 2009; 113(13):2895-901.

[66] Tefferi A. Myelofibrosis with myeloid metaplasia. *N. Engl. J. Med.* 2000; 342:1255–65.

[67] Cervantes F., Pereira A. Prognostication in primary myelofibrosis. *Curr. Hematol. Malig. Rep.* 2012; 7(1): 43-9.

[68] Helbig G, Wieczorkiewicz A, Woźniczka K, Wiśniewska-Piąty K, Rusek A, Kyrcz-Krzemień S. The JAK2V617F tyrosine kinase mutation has no impact on overall survival and the risk of leukemic transformation in myelofibrosis. *Med. Oncol.* 2012. [Epub ahead of print]

[69] Chauffaille ML. Eosinofilia reacional, leucemia eosinofílica crônica e síndrome hipereosinofílica Idiopática. *Rev. bras. Hematol. Hemoter.* 2010; 32:5.

[70] Ljungman P, Bregni M, Brune M, et al. European Group for Blood and Marrow Transplantation. Allogeneic and autologous transplantation for haematological diseases, solid tumours and immune disorders: current practice in Europe 2009. *Bone Marrow Transplant.* 2010;45(2):219-34.

[71] Dupriez B, Morel P, Demory JL, et al. Prognostic factors in agnogenic myeloid metaplasia: a report on 195 cases with a new scoring system. *Blood.* 1996; 88(3):1013-8.

[72] Cervantes F, Barosi G, Demory JL, et al. Myelofibrosis with myeloid metaplasia in young individuals: disease characteristics, prognostic

factors and identification of risk groups. *Br. J. Haematol.* 1998 Aug;102(3):684-90.

[73]   Tefferi A, Huang J, Schwager S, Li CY, Pardanani A, Mesa RA. Validation and comparison of contemporary prognostic models in primary myelofibrosis: analysis based on 334 patients from a single institution. *Cancer.* 2007;109(10):2083-8.

[74]   Passamonti F, Cervantes F, Vannucchi AM, et al. Dynamic International Prognostic Scoring System (DIPSS) predicts progression to acute myeloid leukemia in primary myelofibrosis. *Blood.* 2010;116(15):2857-8.

[75]   Gangat N, Caramazza D, Vaidya R, et al. DIPSS plus: a refined Dynamic International Prognostic Scoring System for primary myelofibrosis that incorporates prognostic information from karyotype, platelet count, and transfusion status. *J. Clin. Oncol.* 2011;29(4):392-7.

[76]   Elliott MA, Verstovsek S, Dingli D, et al. Monocytosis is an adverse prognostic factor for survival in younger patients with primary myelofibrosis. *Leuk. Res.* 2007; 31(11):1503-9.

[77]   Vardiman JW, Brunning RD, Harris NL: WHO histological classification of chronic myeloproliferative diseases, in Jaffe ES, Harris NL, Stein H, et al (eds): World Health Organization classification of tumors: Tumours of the haematopoietic and lymphoid tissues. Lyon, France, International Agency for Research on Cancer Press, 2001, 17-44.

[78]   Hussein K, Huang J., Lasho T, et al. Karyotype complements the International Prognostic Scoring System for primary myelofibrosis. *Eur. J. Haematol.* 2009; 82(4):255-9.

[79]   Shaffer LG, Slovak ML, Campbel LJ (eds). ISCN 2009 - An International System for Human Cytogenetic Nomeclature. S. Karger, Basel, 2009.

[80]   Vannucchi AM. Management of myelofibrosis. *Hematology Am. Soc. Hematol. Educ. Program.* 2011; 222-30.

[81]   Tefferi A, Murphy S. Current opinion in essential thrombocythemia: pathogenesis, diagnosis, and management. *Blood Rev.* 2001;15(3):121-31.

[82]   Barbui T, Thiele J, Vannucchi AM, Tefferi A. Problems and pitfalls regarding WHO-defined diagnosis of early/prefibrotic primary myelofibrosis versus essential thrombocythemia. *Leukemia.* 2013;27(10):1953-8.

[83] Mascarenhas J, Mughal TI, Verstovsek S. Biology and Clinical Management of Myeloproliferative Neoplasms and Development of the JAK Inhibitor Ruxolitinib. *Curr. Med. Chem.* 2012;19(26):4399-413.

[84] Rotunno G, Mannarelli C, Guglielmelli P, Pacilli A, Pancrazzi A, Pieri L, et al. Impact of Calreticulin Mutations on Clinical and Hematological Phenotype and Outcome in Essential Thrombocythemia. *Blood.* 2013.

[85] Buhr T, Hebeda K, Kaloutsi V, Porwit A, Van der Walt J, Kreipe H. European Bone Marrow Working Group trial on reproducibility of World Health Organization criteria to discriminate essential thrombocythemia from prefibrotic primary myelofibrosis. *Haematologica.* 2012;97(3):360-5.

[86] Wilkins BS, Erber WN, Bareford D, Buck G, Wheatley K, East CL, et al. Bone marrow pathology in essential thrombocythemia: interobserver reliability and utility for identifying disease subtypes. *Blood.* 2008; 111(1):60-70.

[87] Mignon I, Grand F, Boyer F, Hunault-Berger M, Hamel JF, Macchi L. Thrombin generation and procoagulant phospholipids in patients with essential thrombocythemia and reactive thrombocytosis. *Am. J. Hematol.* 2013;88(12):1007-11.

[88] Barbui T, Thiele J, Carobbio A, Guglielmelli P, Rambaldi A, Vannucchi AM, et al. Discriminating between essential thrombocythemia and masked polycythemia vera in JAK2 mutated patients. *Am. J. Hematol.* 2014.

[89] Girodon F, Bonicelli G, Schaeffer C, Mounier M, Carillo S, Lafon I, et al. Significant increase in the apparent incidence of essential thrombocythemia related to new WHO diagnostic criteria: a population-based study. *Haematologica.* 2009;94(6):865-9.

[90] Geyer HL, Emanuel RM, Dueck AC, Kiladjian JJ, Xiao Z, Slot S, et al. Distinct clustering of symptomatic burden amongst myeloproliferative neoplasm patients: retrospective assessment in 1470 patients. *Blood.* 2014.

[91] Scherber R, Dueck AC, Johansson P, Barbui T, Barosi G, Vannucchi AM, et al. The Myeloproliferative Neoplasm Symptom Assessment Form (MPN-SAF): international prospective validation and reliability trial in 402 patients. *Blood.* 2011;118(2):401-8.

[92] Cervantes F. Management of essential thrombocythemia. *Hematology Am. Soc. Hematol. Educ. Program.* 2011;2011:215-21.

[93] Passamonti F, Thiele J, Girodon F, Rumi E, Carobbio A, Gisslinger H, et al. A prognostic model to predict survival in 867 World Health

Organization-defined essential thrombocythemia at diagnosis: a study by the International Working Group on Myelofibrosis Research and Treatment. *Blood*. 2012;120(6):1197-201.

[94]   Barbui T, Thiele J, Passamonti F, Rumi E, Boveri E, Ruggeri M, et al. Survival and disease progression in essential thrombocythemia are significantly influenced by accurate morphologic diagnosis: an international study. *J. Clin. Oncol.* 2011;29(23):3179-84.

[95]   Campbell PJ, MacLean C, Beer PA, Buck G, Wheatley K, Kiladjian JJ, et al. Correlation of blood counts with vascular complications in essential thrombocythemia: analysis of the prospective PT1 cohort. *Blood*. 2012;120(7):1409-11.

[96]   Chou YS, Gau JP, Yu YB, Pai JT, Hsiao LT, Liu JH, et al. Leukocytosis in polycythemia vera and splenomegaly in essential thrombocythemia are independent risk factors for hemorrhage. *Eur. J. Haematol.* 2013;90(3):228-36.

[97]   Montanaro M, Latagliata R, Cedrone M, Spadea A, Rago A, Di Giandomenico J, et al. Thrombosis and survival in essential thrombocythemia: A regional study of 1144 patients. *Am. J. Hematol.* 2014.

[98]   Alvarez-Larrán A, Bellosillo B, Pereira A, Kerguelen A, Hernández-Boluda JC, Martínez-Avilés L, et al. JAK2V617F monitoring in polycythemia vera and essential thrombocythemia: clinical usefulness for predicting myelofibrotic transformation and thrombotic events. *Am. J. Hematol.* 2014.

[99]   Sever M, Newberry KJ, Verstovsek S. Therapeutic options for patients with polycythemia vera and essential thrombocythemia refractory/resistant to hydroxyurea. *Leuk. Lymphoma*. 2014.

[100] Hernández-Boluda JC, Pereira A, Cervantes F, Gómez M, Arellano-Rodrigo E, Alvarez-Larrán A, et al. Clinical evaluation of the European LeukemiaNet response criteria in patients with essential thrombocythemia treated with anagrelide. *Ann. Hematol.* 2013;92(6): 771-5.

[101] Gugliotta L, Besses C, Griesshammer M, Harrison C, Kiladjian JJ, Coll R, et al. Combination therapy of hydroxycarbamide with anagrelide inpatients with essential thrombocythemia in the evaluation of Xagrid(R): efficacy and long-term safety study. *Haematologica*. 2013.

[102] Wolf D, Rudzki J, Gastl G. Current treatment concepts of Philadelphia-negative MPN. *Curr. Cancer Drug Targets*. 2011;11(1):44-55.

[103] Gisslinger H, Gotic M, Holowiecki J, Penka M, Thiele J, Kvasnicka HM, et al. Anagrelide compared with hydroxyurea in WHO-classified essential thrombocythemia: the ANAHYDRET Study, a randomized controlled trial. *Blood.* 2013;121(10):1720-8.

[104] Souza, MC., Rodrigues, CA, Silva, M.R R, Ribeiro, J, Tognon, R, Castro, FA, Simões, BP, Souto, EX, Chauffaille, ML. Application of five prognostic survival scores to primary myelofibrosis in 62 Brazilian patients. *Med Oncol.* 2013. 30:555.

INDEX

C

D

E

F

G

H

N

O

P

Q

R

S

symptoms, vii, viii, ix, 3, 8, 10, 11, 13, 16, 19, 20, 22, 23, 24, 25, 28, 47, 55, 57, 58, 60, 62, 63, 67, 100, 102, 103, 107, 108, 109, 110, 111, 113, 115, 116, 117
syndrome, ix, 11, 18, 19, 22, 23, 27, 35, 40, 47, 49, 72, 73, 78, 100, 101, 122
synthesis, 22, 29
systemic mastocytosis, vii, 101

T

T cell, 22, 58
T lymphocytes, 32, 50
tachycardia, 29
target, x, 13, 80, 90, 92, 94, 101
techniques, 2, 103
temperature, 58
testing, 50, 63, 64, 67
TGF, 15, 16
therapeutic approaches, 91, 93
therapeutic use, 37
therapeutics, 72
therapy, ix, x, 4, 6, 7, 13, 14, 18, 20, 24, 29, 33, 34, 37, 45, 46, 47, 51, 54, 64, 72, 76, 92, 101, 102, 104, 105, 106, 110, 111, 115, 116, 117, 120, 121, 126
thorium, 15
thrombin, 113
thrombocytopenia, 17, 21, 23, 27, 53, 64, 65, 104, 110, 111
thrombocytosis, viii, ix, 8, 12, 14, 17, 22, 24, 26, 27, 51, 54, 55, 57, 58, 60, 64, 68, 100, 101, 103, 104, 111, 112, 113, 116, 122, 125
thrombo-hemorrhagic complications, vii
thrombopoietin, 49, 50, 58, 71, 106, 107
thrombosis, x, 4, 7, 10, 11, 14, 25, 26, 27, 28, 29, 36, 51, 52, 53, 58, 60, 70, 101, 108, 114, 116
thymine, 106
thyroid, 79, 96
tissue, 5, 27, 67, 105
tobacco, 25
toluene, 38
toxicity, 7, 53

transcription, 66, 80
transcripts, 3, 6, 31, 33, 35
transformation, vii, 2, 8, 11, 24, 27, 28, 42, 48, 51, 52, 53, 80, 93, 104, 107, 108, 114, 116, 119, 120, 123, 126
transforming growth factor, 39
transfusion, 20, 23, 42, 44, 46, 111, 124
transient ischemic attack, 25, 58, 113
translocation, viii, ix, 2, 3, 5, 39, 64, 66, 72, 75, 76, 78, 80, 84, 89, 94, 96, 97, 102
transplant, 21, 22, 46, 91, 110, 115
transplantation, 7, 8, 9, 20, 34, 44, 45, 46, 92, 105, 121, 123
transport, 78
trauma, 27
treatment, vii, viii, ix, 2, 6, 7, 10, 18, 19, 20, 22, 24, 26, 28, 29, 36, 37, 38, 39, 40, 46, 47, 49, 50, 51, 53, 54, 63, 69, 72, 90, 91, 92, 93, 94, 96, 100, 101, 102, 103, 104, 105, 106, 107, 108, 110, 115, 116, 117, 119, 120, 121, 126
trial, 29, 46, 47, 48, 122, 125, 127
trisomy, 4, 56, 66, 107
trisomy 21, 56, 66
tryptophan, 107
tumo(u)r, 23, 47, 123
tumor necrosis factor, 23, 47
tumors, 19, 83, 89, 124
turnover, 11
tyrosine, ix, 2, 6, 33, 34, 42, 76, 79, 80, 96, 100, 102, 105, 118, 119, 121, 123
Tyrosine, 6, 122

U

UK, 29
ultrasound, 51
United States, 2, 24

V

validation, 53, 125
valine, 106
variables, 40, 41, 43, 48, 110

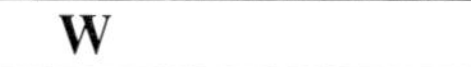

W